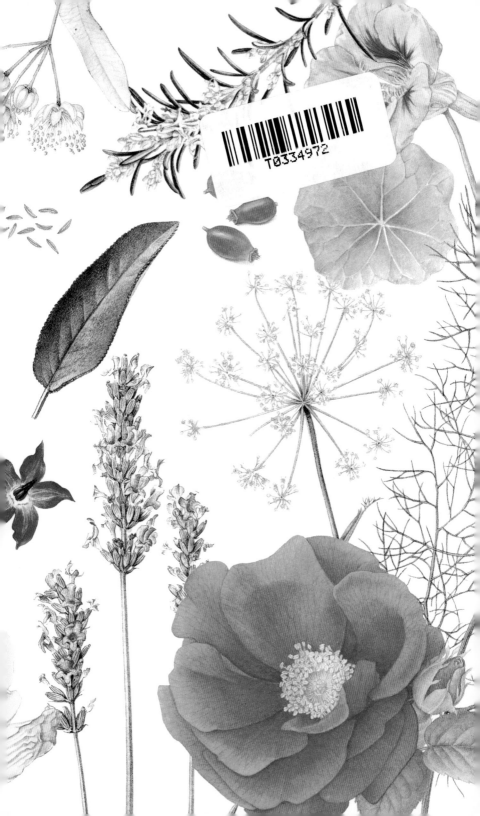

T0334972

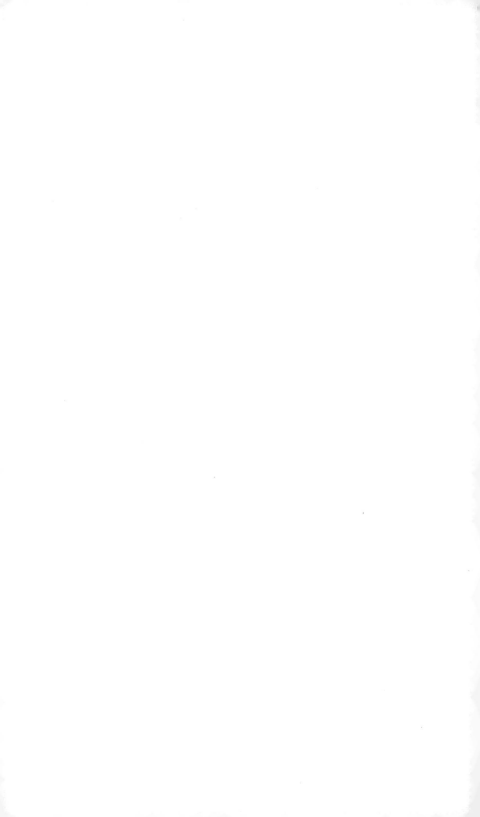

The
Herbal
Year

CHRISTINA HART-DAVIES

The Herbal Year

Folklore, History & Remedies

YALE UNIVERSITY PRESS
New Haven and London

Every effort has been made to include formal citation of copyright material – any necessary amendments will be taken into future printings.

For information about this and other Yale University Press publications, please contact:
U.S. Office: sales.press@yale.edu yalebooks.com
Europe Office: sales@yaleup.co.uk yalebooks.co.uk

Designed and set in Joanna Nova by Tetragon, London
Printed in China

Library of Congress Control Number: 2023946544

ISBN 978-0-300-26586-6

A catalogue record for this book is available from the British Library.

10 9 8 7 6 5 4 3 2 1

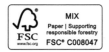

Contents

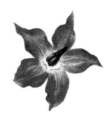

Disclaimer

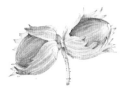

Neither the author nor the publisher of this book is a medical or health professional, and the book is not intended to provide medical advice or treatment. The information on herbs and herbal remedies is provided for informational and historical purposes only and is based on the author's research and personal experiences, not on any clinical or medical expertise or investigation. It is not meant as a substitute for medical advice or as an endorsement of the safety or efficacy of herbs for the uses described. Your use of this information is at your own discretion and risk. In addition, some herbs can cause allergic reactions or interfere or react with other medications in a harmful way. Always consult with your physician or healthcare provider before taking any new medication, herbal or otherwise. Never consume any herbs if you are pregnant or have a medical condition without first checking with your physician or healthcare provider.

The author has made every effort to ensure the book is as accurate as possible, based on historical and commonly known uses of herbs, but it may contain errors, omissions or material that is out of date by the time you read it. Neither the author nor the publisher have any legal responsibility or liability for errors, omissions or out-of-date material or for the reader's use or application of the information included in the book.

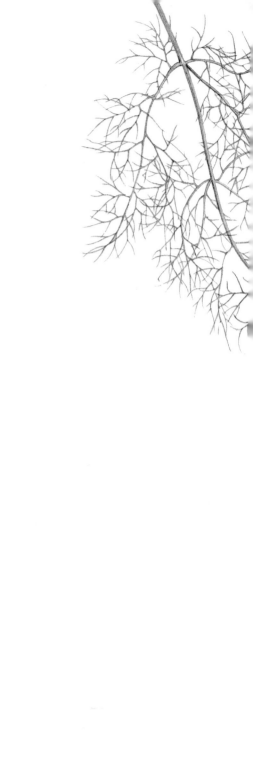

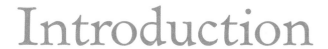

Introduction

Hence sprang the art of medicine.
Such things alone had Nature
decreed should be our remedies,
provided everywhere, easy to discover
and costing nothing – the things
in fact that support our life.

PLINY THE ELDER,
Natural History (c.77 CE)

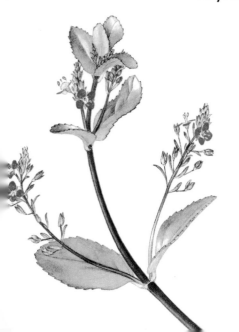

his book, though by no means comprehensive, tells the stories of some of our commonest medicinal plants through the year, with comments from writers who have studied and used them down the ages. Though folk medicine is practised worldwide, the main focus here is on herbs growing wild in Europe and North America. Many of the plants described can be grown in temperate gardens anywhere.

A brief history of herbal medicine

Our prehistoric ancestors must have been the first herbalists. Animals, including primates, have been observed apparently self-medicating, and in early man this instinctive behaviour must have developed into conscious choice. Concentrated deposits of pollen from yarrow, chamomile and other medicinal herbs have been found in a Neanderthal burial dating from over 50,000 years ago, suggesting that our nearest relatives may have collected such herbs for ritual or therapeutic purposes. We have no direct evidence for this, of course – not even any cave paintings. When early *Homo sapiens* ventured into the sacred inner caves, pigments in hand, he depicted the animals he hunted or admired or feared, but never the plants they all depended upon. Depictions of plants do not appear anywhere until about the time agriculture began. Throughout history, pain and illness were the norm, and some people would have become experts in alleviating these, perhaps supported by their community as they concentrated on the task of healing. These were the medicine men, the shamans, the wise women, the healers found in every society.

Not until writing began do we glimpse any concrete evidence of herbal therapy. The Ramesseum papyri, a collection of ancient Egyptian medical texts from the nineteenth century BCE are the oldest yet found. Ayurvedic and Chinese medicine had both been flourishing for centuries before their earliest extant texts were written. The earliest western records come from classical Greece. So the oral traditions of medicine, practised all over the world since the beginning, were finally recorded in writing in certain cultures.

We know of some early scholars and physicians from their surviving writings or from references to them in later manuscripts. We know that Hippocrates (c.460–c.375 BCE), for example, brought a rational approach to medicine, using observation, diagnosis, skilled surgery and wholistic treatment. In the fourth century BCE, the Greek scholar Theophrastus wrote a meticulously researched treatise describing plants, their cultivation and uses. In Rome, Pliny the Elder, who died investigating the eruption of Vesuvius in 79 CE, wrote his monumental *Natural History*, several volumes of which describe plants and herbal medicine. His near-contemporary, Dioscorides, a Greek doctor working for the Roman army, wrote *De Materia Medica*, which remained a trusted textbook for about 1,500 years. It included some five hundred therapeutic herbs. We also know of around fifty women physicians working in Ancient Greece and Rome, treating more than just obstetric and gynaecological conditions.

In the second century CE, Galen wrote a medical manual which developed Hippocrates' idea of humours. These were: blood, phlegm, black bile and yellow bile, each of which was associated with two of the four qualities of heat, coldness, wetness or dryness. Blood, for example, was hot and wet, while yellow bile was hot and dry. Some physicians even included the four seasons, the four elements and even four ages of Man in their diagnostic system. Humours, if out of balance, would cause illness. So herbs were selected to re-establish that balance. This idea persisted for centuries, until, in the sixteenth century, Paracelsus, a Swiss physician, encouraged doctors to rely less on authoritative texts and more on experience and observation. He insisted upon close attention to dosage, echoing Theophrastus, who had written that poisonous thorn apple could make a man 'merely sportive and thinking himself a fine fellow'; or send him permanently insane; or kill him – all

The spotted leaves of lungwort, *Pulmonaria* spp, reminded physicians of diseased lungs, so they used it to treat lung conditions.

depending on the dose taken. Paracelsus also revived and promoted the old idea of the Doctrine of Signatures, which suggested that the Creator had put signs on plants to show which conditions they could be used to treat. It would have been a useful system, if it had worked. Then, only a century or so later, everything changed when the invention of microscopy brought germs to light.

The classical writers all knew and quoted from their predecessors' works, and their manuscripts were copied over and over again. As well as descriptions, many included illustrations to aid identification – after all, mistakes could be fatal. Pliny critically remarked: 'for paintings, you know, are deceitful', as they often show only one stage of a plant's growth. While early illustrations (such as those credited to Cratevas in the first century BCE) were accurate, and probably drawn from life, as time went on the paintings became degraded copies of copies of copies. By the tenth century in Europe, many illustrations were more about decoration than information – perhaps it was assumed that everyone knew the plants described in the text. A copy of Dioscorides' *De Materia Medica* was written and beautifully illustrated in Constantinople in about 512 CE. It was originally made as a luxury gift for an imperial princess, but ended up being used for centuries as a textbook in the hospital of a Constantinople monastery. There is a record of a physician, Nathanael, paying for its rebinding in 1406. Known as the *Codex Vindobonensis*, today it is a UNESCO heritage treasure, kept in the National Library in Vienna.

Post-Roman Britain (from about 400 CE) is usually represented as a country sunk in the Dark Ages, brutish and ignorant. But in fact, learning, not least on medical matters, continued throughout this period. Texts and fragments of manuscript were collated and copied, though there appear to have been few ground-breaking new theories. The tenth-century *Leechbook of Bald* and *Lacnunga* were both collections of medical writings and included passages from classical authors, alongside more home-grown 'leechcraft'. Incidentally, 'leech' (*laece*) was the Old English word for a doctor, and the same word, by a completely different etymology, also meant the blood-sucking creature employed for blood-letting treatments. To confuse matters even further, the Old English word *lic*, meaning 'body' (alive or dead) was pronounced in almost the same way.

We underestimate the amount of international travel and trade there was even in early times. Scholars journeyed between courts, monasteries and medical schools, taking manuscripts, herbs and medicines with them. All monasteries had extensive gardens, growing food, medicines and herbs for strewing. After a warm period lasting about four hundred years, in the fourteenth century the European climate turned colder and wetter, so that plants that originated in warmer places became harder to grow. However, it has been estimated that by 1500 around three hundred different herbs were still being grown in Britain, as opposed to being imported in dried form.

After the fall of the Roman Empire, medical scholarship flourished in the Middle East, with the translation of classical Greek and Latin texts, and with new books being researched and written. In the eleventh century, the Persian polymath known as Avicenna published a medical text that would remain influential for generations. In the early twelfth century, Muslim botanist and physician Ibn al-Suri is recorded as plant-hunting in Lebanon accompanied by a botanical illustrator. This scholarship sparked a European revival in medical learning, and herbal manuscripts flooded into monasteries and the newly founded universities.

But things really took off with the invention of printing, and in the 1500s new printed herbals became generally available. Soon, even modest households would have a Bible, a Prayer Book and a herbal on their bookshelf, if nothing else. The best known is John Gerard's *Herbal*, published in 1597. It is comprehensive (running to almost 1,500 pages), engagingly written and illustrated with botanically accurate woodcuts. Based on an earlier Flemish herbal, it includes plants from the author's own garden in London, and some plants newly introduced from the Americas: the first published European illustration of the potato appears in Gerard's *Herbal*. Many printed herbals by other writers followed over the years – notably one by Nicholas Culpeper in 1652, which was reprinted many times. In 1872, Francis Kilvert, a curate in the Welsh borders, had a conversation with an elderly parishioner about the local names and the uses of some wild plants. Kilvert's diary entry concludes: 'The old man's work was done, he put up his tools, took me home with him, and lent me Culpeper's *Herbal*.' Editions of Culpeper and Gerard are still in print today, probably the best known among the many such books printed since. Perhaps the most comprehensive herbal in recent times is Maud Grieve's *A Modern Herbal*, published in 1931.

Many writers had firm opinions
and were not afraid to express
them in print. Gerard scorned what
he saw as superstitions; Culpeper railed
against the medical establishment of
his day; while Dr John Hill, in his
1756 herbal, took every opportunity
to criticise Linnaeus's classifications
of plants. It makes for entertaining reading, along
with the best herbal advice of the time. Many writers,
stretching right back to Theophrastus, wanted to tell
people about simple remedies they could find for themselves,
instead of paying physicians for complicated, expensive ones.

The oral tradition continued alongside the written,
scholarly one; sometimes they were in competition,
sometimes they learned from each other. Most of the
published writers were men, while, in Europe at least, the oral
and informal tradition was mainly women's work. We have
little evidence of early 'folk medicine', other than references
in plays, songs, proverbs and rhymes. Most households of
any size kept a 'household book' in which they noted down
recipes, household hints and remedies. These books were
passed down through generations and a few still survive. In
the twentieth century, researchers began recording people's –
especially old people's – memories of natural medicine. There
is an encouraging continuity through the ages: a Scottish
granny treated a child's scalded face with an ointment made
from ivy leaves – just as the Anglo-Saxons did, and the
Romans before them. There are also interesting geographical
parallels: for example, the Mahuna in America found that

the bark of a Californian oak species would stop bleeding, while in Britain we used our native oak for the same effect. Colonisation and trade introduced new medicinal plants to Europe, while Europeans exported some of theirs – along with their illnesses, of course. Now most herbs can be grown anywhere the climate allows, or bought in preserved form.

Without the benefit of our modern scientific knowledge, diseases must have been perplexing, even appearing supernatural to our ancestors. So it is not surprising that medicine sometimes became entangled with magic and superstition. It is not that our forebears were stupid: they were intelligent people, doing their best with the experience, observation, tradition and information available at the time. And their efforts were not always wide of the mark: recent research at Nottingham University into an Anglo-Saxon treatment for an eye infection (a stye) found that each of the ingredients by themselves had some small effect; but combined and prepared exactly as instructed, they would destroy the MRSA bacteria as effectively as today's standard conventional medication.

As scientific practice grew in the seventeenth and eighteenth centuries, so botany and medicine began to diverge, and herbal remedies came to be abandoned by many as unscientific, superstitious nonsense. In 1756, John Hill lamented that 'chemistry has banished natural medicines'. Nineteenth-century advances in medical science included better training for doctors and the rise of bacteriology, pharmacology, sanitisation and vaccination, while a 'change of air' and regular purging remained fashionably popular among the public. As ever, there was unscrupulous peddling of quack remedies to the gullible, advertised in newspapers and magazines of the time.

In *Cider with Rosie*, describing his Gloucestershire childhood in the 1920s, Laurie Lee reminds us how frequent serious illness was, especially among the poor. Children faded quickly and often parents could do little but 'burn coal-tar and pray'. He himself often fell ill with dangerous fevers, and was dosed with 'a hell-draught of unspeakable vileness'. However, many country people continued to use familiar plants as they always had, supplementing – or sometimes replacing – costly drugs. There is plenty of anecdotal evidence for the use of common plants to treat injuries and everyday ailments at this time. Some of these home remedies are described in the following chapters. They are mentioned for historical interest and are not suggestions for self-medication. You should always consult your doctor about any symptoms or conditions you have and should discuss herbal remedies with qualified experts before using them, especially if you are pregnant, trying to get pregnant or are nursing.

Pharmaceutical medicines were largely manufactured from plants, and at the start of the twentieth century Britain imported many of its drugs and raw materials from Germany. So, when the First World War began, the British Board of Agriculture hurriedly issued lists of medicinal plants to be grown or foraged in Britain. Herbs such as feverfew, tansy, comfrey and greater celandine were already grown commercially, but others were needed. Market gardens started growing more herbs, and Maud Grieve, the herbalist and writer, set up a large herb farm in Buckinghamshire, staffed by Belgian refugees. Similar measures came into force during the Second World War, and in 1941 the Vegetable Drugs Committee was established to oversee the growing and collecting of plants. National Rose Hip Syrup was made with rose hips collected from hedgerows by the general public. It kept children supplied with vitamin C when the import of citrus fruits became well-nigh impossible.

Although most of our conventional drugs originated from plants, the constituents are now synthesised. Since the 1970s there has been a revival of interest in natural treatments, echoing a desire to be more self-sufficient and reconnected with nature. As Anthony Huxley wrote in 1984, 'green medicine is being born again'. A new respect for traditional medicine is even growing among the medical profession. My own doctor recommended arnica for extensive bruising, and the NHS now uses honey-impregnated dressings for intractable leg ulcers, just as Theophrastus recommended in ancient Greece over 2,300 years ago.

∾ Using herbs safely

This book, while not comprehensive, tells the stories of some of the commonest medicinal plants throughout the year, with comments from many of the writers mentioned above. It is intended to provide some historical context for many of the herbs and herbal remedies still used by many today, but it is not a treatise on herbal medicine nor should it be read as an endorsement of the safety or efficacy of herbs to treat any of the ailments or conditions described. It is not intended to provide guidance for any particular use of herbs or course of treatment.

Though folk medicine is practised worldwide, the main focus here is on Europe and North America. Most of the wild plants described can be grown in temperate gardens anywhere. Always take care when collecting herbs in the countryside. If you go foraging for wild herbs, be sure to take a reliable identification guide with you and observe local laws on collecting plant material. Herbs can easily be confused and some plants, of course, can be harmful or poisonous.

The use of herbs is not without risk. Individuals may be allergic to particular plants, and some herbs can interact negatively with other herbs or medications and may be dangerous with certain medical conditions. It is important before beginning to use any herb or herbal treatment that you consult a physician or other qualified professional. This is especially important if you are pregnant, trying to get pregnant or are nursing. The book includes a few of my own simple recipes to make at home. While it can be fun making 'simples', these are my own recipes, drawn from historical sources, and have not been tested in any scientific way. If you choose to make them, care should be taken and they should be used at your own risk. These home recipes are not cures or treatments for any medical ailments or conditions. The proper dosing of herbs can depend on a number of factors such as the quality and origin of the herb and the age, weight and overall health of the individual. Again, it is always safest before beginning to use any herbal treatment to consult with an expert or qualified professional.

Eyebrights, *Euphrasia* spp,
were used for eye conditions.

❧ What is a herb?

To a botanist, a herb is any plant without a woody stem.
To a cook, it is a plant that enhances flavours. While to a
herbalist, it is one that promotes health and well-being.
Plants may have different amounts of bioactive compounds
(and therefore healing effects), depending on such factors as
their maturity, the weather, the habitat and the soil in which
they grow – even the time of day when they are picked.
Experienced herbalists would take account of all these
factors and search out the best plants to use. Great care was
taken with dosage, as many healing plants can be toxic, too.
Alarmingly, the Greek word *pharmakon* meant both 'medicine'
and 'poison'.

Sometimes the whole herb was used in one treatment.
Various parts of the plant might be given separately – the
leaves and flowers, the fruits, seeds or roots, or even the
bark – and each part may have a different effect. The
vitamin and mineral-rich fruits of raspberry, for example,
are recommended in some modern British herbals to help
treat anaemia, and in China to treat kidney problems.
Meanwhile an infusion of raspberry leaves was traditionally
given both by European and Native American healers to
ease childbirth.

Most of today's drugs originated in plants, and new plant-
based drugs are being discovered all the time: a commonly
used new treatment for some cancers is derived from a
species of *Taxus* (yew) and has the brand name Taxol. The
'active principle' is isolated and nowadays synthesised
in a laboratory. However, herbalists point to the

wisdom of using the whole plant, as it often contains other compounds that alleviate side effects. Aspirin (acetylsalicylic acid), historically derived from willow and meadowsweet, is a case in point: isolated, these salicylates can cause gastric bleeding, but meadowsweet itself also contains soothing, viscous mucilage and tannins which protect the stomach.

Until quite recently the line between food and medicine was less clear. Country people ate wild foods to supplement what they could grow or buy, incidentally improving their health. When diets were limited, leaves could provide missing minerals and trace elements. For example, in the seventeenth century brooklime and scurvy grass were sought out to prevent scurvy (vitamin C deficiency), while in spring various young shoots were eaten to cleanse the blood after a stodgy winter diet. This tradition continues today. In Armenia and Greece I have met old women out on the hillsides collecting leaves for the pot.

∾ Preserving and preparations

People have always found ways to preserve plants for use out of season. Drying is the simplest method. Nicholas Culpeper's advice is still sound: 'Choose only such as are green and full of juice, pick them carefully, and cast away such as are declining, for they will putrefy the rest.' Flowers should be gathered 'at their prime'. Make sure they are dry, shake off any insects, tie in loose bunches and hang in a warm, airy place. I sometimes put them in the airing cupboard with

15

the door slightly open. Once they are dry, strip off the leaves (or chop, if you want to use the stems, too) and put into a clean glass jar. Don't forget to label it. They will keep longer if stored in the dark. Culpeper said that when their colour and scent had gone, so had their 'virtue', or healing powers.

Freshly gathered herbs such as parsley can be chopped and put into the freezer in labelled bags. Roots, usually dug in the autumn, should be cleaned of all soil before drying. Be aware that it is illegal to dig up any wild plant in Britain without the landowner's permission. Similar restrictions may apply elsewhere. Some popular herbs are threatened with extinction due to over-collection in the wild. Better to grow your own or buy from reputable, licensed growers. Some herbs advertised on the internet may be adulterated with cheaper additives; so, again, buy from trusted sources.

Herbs can be preserved in other ways, too. Some of the more popular preparations are described below. Extracts and distillations are made commercially from some herbs, but this cannot really be done at home. They are much stronger than the preparations described below, so do heed the warnings given. Throughout this book there are recipes I use to treat some of my own minor ailments. These home recipes work for me, but are not cures or treatments for any medical conditions. You should always consult a medical professional about your own symptoms before using any herbal remedy, and for persistent or serious conditions you should, of course, always seek medical help. Preparing home remedies follows a very long tradition, reconnects us with the natural world and brings an empowering sense of self-care.

* A **simple** is a remedy made using only one herb.
* An **infusion** is also called a 'tea' or 'tisane'. Pour boiling water onto fresh or dried herbs in a cup or a teapot, cover and allow to infuse for several minutes, then strain. Or you could use a tea-infuser. The volatile oils in the leaves or flowers will evaporate if the vessel isn't covered.
* **Decoctions** are made by simmering herbs in water for some time and then straining through a fine sieve (strainer) before bottling. This method is especially useful for hard material, such as roots or bark. Decoctions will keep for two to three days and are either taken neat or diluted with hot water.
* A **compress** is a clean cloth soaked in an infusion or decoction and applied hot to the affected part, with care taken not to scald the skin. It should be bandaged firmly in place and replaced when it cools.
* A **poultice** is when the hot plant itself is applied, either wrapped in gauze or applied direct to the skin. It is used in the same way as a compress.
* A **syrup** starts as a strong, reduced decoction, to which honey or sugar is added. It is then simmered, with constant stirring, until the right consistency is reached. Then it is bottled and labelled. Syrups will keep for two weeks to several months, depending on the ratio of sugar to liquid.
* For a **culinary vinegar**, fresh herbs or whole spices are steeped in vinegar in the dark for at least two weeks, during which the jar should be shaken daily. The vinegar is then

strained and bottled. For a gift, make the vinegar with fresh herbs and then add a decorative sprig of dried herb to the bottle: that way the herb will keep its shape better.

* For a **medicinal vinegar**, the ratio of chopped fresh herb to vinegar is much higher than for culinary vinegar. The herbs are steeped in vinegar in the dark for two weeks; the jar should be shaken daily. Once strained and bottled, the vinegar will keep for several months and is usually used diluted.

* **Tinctures** are made with chopped fresh or dried herbs steeped in alcohol for two weeks, then strained and squeezed before bottling. Tinctures will keep indefinitely and are usually used diluted.

* **Flavoured oils** are made in the same way as culinary vinegar, above, using a very lightly flavoured oil as a base. They make attractive gifts.

* **Infused oils** are made by gently heating together fresh or dried herbs and oil. This can be done in the sun over a long time, or in a bain-marie (water bath) more quickly. Once poured into a clean, dark glass bottle, an infused oil should keep for up to a year. It can be used as it is, or made into other preparations, as below.

* A **liniment** is a mixture of an infused oil and a herb tincture.

* A **salve** or balm is made with 4 parts of infused oil to 1 part of pure beeswax warmed in a bain-marie (water bath).

* **Ointments** are made in the same way as salves, but using 10 parts of infused oil to 1 part of beeswax. They should not be used on inflamed or broken skin. Ointments can also be made with any fat that will solidify on its own, such as cocoa butter or coconut oil, or even lard. An Anglo-Saxon herbal

even recommended boiling ivy leaves in butter to make an ointment for sunburn.

❧ A note on weights and measures

Both imperial and metric weights and measures are given, when appropriate, in the recipes in this book.

From the beginning, mixing of ingredients was often relatively informal, with texts specifying 'a handful' or 'a three-finger pinch' and 'enough water to cover'. Instructions like 'enough dried herb to cover a penny' were common. In medicine, dosage can be extremely important, so for more precise measurements, apothecaries used standardised weights. For many centuries in Britain there were three different systems, all based on the *grain*, the weight of a specified number of dry grains of wheat. In the *Apothecaries'* system, twenty grains made a *scruple*, three scruples made a *dram*, eight drams made an *ounce* and twelve ounces made a *pound*. This differs from the *Troy* and *Avoirdupois* (imperial) systems.

The term *pennyweight*, used in the Troy system, meant exactly that: the weight of a penny coin. An English silver penny was minted to weigh a standard number of grains. The dram derives from the ancient Greek coin the drachma, as suggested by its old spelling 'drachm'. In Britain, the dram was also a measure of volume, properly called a 'fluid dram'. And 'dram' remains an affectionate term for a small tot of alcohol.

Instructions in old herbals to stir a mixture while reciting a prayer three times may be more than just superstition or a wish to heal the soul, as well as the body. In the absence of clocks or watches, it was a good way of judging a length of time. It still works: weren't we all, during the pandemic, encouraged to wash our hands while singing 'Happy Birthday to You' twice?

The proper time to gather a particular herb was often expressed in astronomical terms: 'at the rising of Arcturus' or 'just after the solstice', for example. However, more agricultural terms – such as 'when the rye is ripening' – were probably more useful, as they reflected weather conditions in any year. If the rye was ripening early, your herb would be ready early, too.

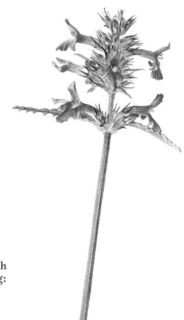

Betony, *Betonica officinalis*, was considered such a valuable remedy that the Romans had a saying: 'Sell your coat and buy betony!'

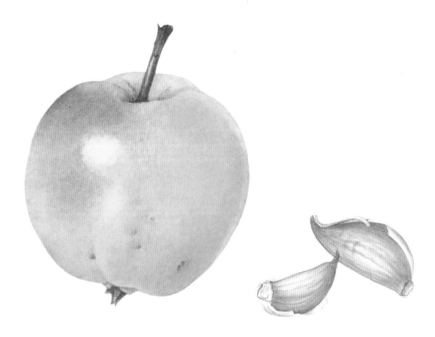

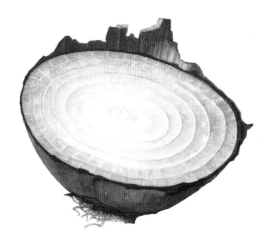

Foods
as medicine

Let food be your medicine

HIPPOCRATES
(c.460–c.375 BCE)

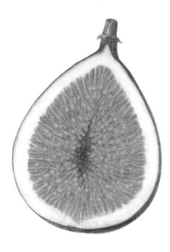

The aphorism attributed to Hippocrates, the ancient Greek 'Father of Medicine', was most likely written by one of his followers who subscribed to the same principles of wholistic healing, where lifestyle and diet were as important as medication. He recognised that, as many illnesses may be caused or exacerbated by dietary factors, the right foods could act as remedies.

Until the mid-twentieth century doctors were expensive, and so poorer people did the best they could with whatever came to hand. And there was a body of oral tradition to draw upon: your grandmother knew what you should eat when you were constipated or needed a tonic. People knew that cabbage leaves, blanched in boiling water and wrapped around a sprained or painful joint, would relieve discomfort. Everyone reached for honey and lemon to soothe a sore throat and help with a cough. Honey is both antiseptic and expectorant, so they were right.

Some commodities, commonplace as foods elsewhere, were employed as home remedies in Britain. In the 1950s, olive oil was an exotic substance bought from the chemist's in a small bottle with square shoulders. It was warmed in front of the fire and then dripped into our ears to soften hard wax when we had earache. Nowadays olive oil is readily available for cooking, too, and is considered a good ingredient of a healthy diet.

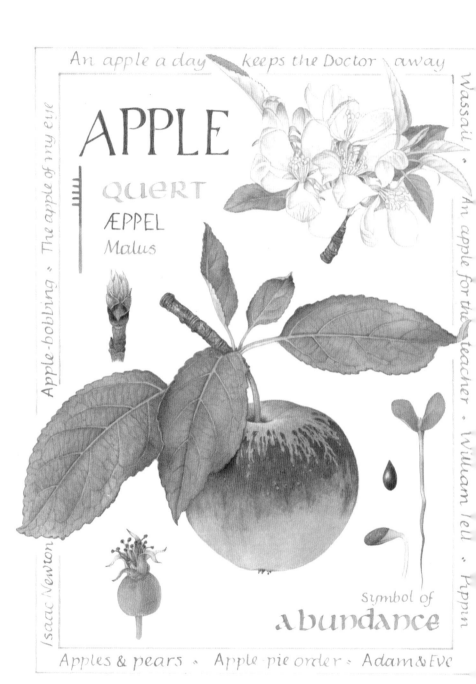

An apple a day   keeps the Doctor   away

Wassail • An apple for the teacher • William Tell • Pippin

APPLE

QUERT

ÆPPEL

Malus

Apple-bobbing • The apple of my eye

Isaac Newton

Symbol of
abundance

Apples & pears • Apple-pie order • Adam & Eve

∾ Apple

'An apple a day keeps the doctor away' goes the old saying, and it is indeed a good source of health-giving fibre and vitamin C. Britain's small, sour, native apples (*Malus sylvestris*) were eaten roasted, made into verjuice (a very acidic juice used like vinegar) or used to flavour hot, spiced ale in the popular dish known as 'lamb's wool'. Cultivated apples (*Malus domestica*), are thought to have been introduced to Britain by the Romans. The Roman writer Pliny listed 200 varieties, and today we have at least 7,500 growing in Britain, for eating, cooking or cider-making.

For nearly fifty years, John Chapman (1774–1847) roamed the far west of America, sowing apple pips collected from cider mills. Known as 'Johnny Appleseed', he single-handedly furnished pioneer communities in three states with apple trees and orchards.

The Anglo-Saxons considered the apple to be one of the nine essential herbs. Eating a fresh apple relieved constipation, while astringent verjuice helped to stop diarrhoea. Pulped apple was applied for eye and skin conditions and for rheumatism. Apples, of course, attracted a good deal of folklore, one example being its reputation for curing warts: you would cut an apple in half, rub it on the wart and then bury it. The wart was supposed to disappear as the apple rotted away.

৵ Oats

Oats (*Avena sativa*), a relative latecomer to cultivation in Britain, were probably domesticated from the wild species growing around wheat and rye fields. Highly nutritious, they have more protein than any other grain; and more fat, too, though polyunsaturated – the right kind! Oat bran is water-soluble fibre, good for the digestive tract. The cereal tends to grow best in cool climates and was a valuable crop in northern areas. Dr Johnson famously defined oats as 'a grain, which in England is generally given to horses, but in Scotland supports the people'. A friend told me how her thrifty grandparents in the Scottish Highlands had a 'porridge drawer'. Porridge was poured into this shallow drawer and left to cool and solidify. Later it was cut into squares and eaten as a snack.

However they are eaten, some find oats to provide an excellent nerve tonic, relieving exhaustion and depression, thanks to the alkaloid avenine. The same component causes horses fed on a surfeit of oats to become highly excitable. In humans, excessive consumption may cause a headache at the back of the skull, but normal amounts are generally considered to be perfectly safe.

Oats hold heat well, so are useful for hot compresses. Gerard describes using a heated bag of oats and bay salt to relieve pain: an early equivalent to popping a wheat-bag into the microwave. Oats were used cosmetically, too, to soothe and soften skin conditions even in babies.

I put some oatmeal and dried lavender flowers into a muslin (cheesecloth) bag

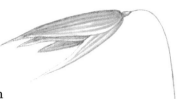

and hang it on the bath tap so
that the water flows through it.
The fragrant bathwater gives my skin
a silky smoothness.

❧ Corn or maize

There is evidence that primitive forms of corn or maize
(*Zea mays*) were cultivated in Mexico around 5500 BCE.
From pre-Columbian times it was grown, together with
beans and squashes, in the 'three sisters' system, an early
example of companion planting. The tall corn provides
something for the beans to climb up; the beans fix nitrogen
in the soil; and the large squash leaves shade the soil and
conserve water. The fruits of the three plants complement
each other nutritionally, too, and can all be dried for winter
use.

Corn is no longer found in the wild, but is cultivated in
tropical and temperate zones everywhere. Fifty per cent of
the world's production is in the USA, mainly in the 'corn
belt' states, and mostly for animal feed. Sweetcorn has always
occurred as a natural mutation in field-corn crops. It was first
given to early settlers by the Iroquois in 1779, and cultivars
were developed in the nineteenth century. People eat various
types of corn fresh, ground into flour, cornmeal or hominy
grits, or made into beer and spirits. They extract oil from
it and even make it into popcorn snacks. The Cherokee,
Mohegan and Tewa also used corn medicinally, mainly for
skin disorders.

Those living on a limited corn-based diet, especially one with no animal proteins, run the risk of niacin (vitamin B3) deficiency, which causes pellagra – a serious condition that leads to dermatitis, diarrhoea and dementia. While corn is rich in vitamin B6, it has very little vitamin B3 in an available form. However, soaking the corn in lye (made from wood ash) or in slaked lime, the traditional Native American way, makes niacin bio-available.

Corn was brought back to Europe by Columbus, and soon spread to Britain, where it was called maize. Gerard grew it in his garden towards the end of the sixteenth century. He thought little of its nutritional value or taste, calling it 'a more convenient food for swine than for man'. Its medicinal value lay particularly in 'cornsilk', the long styles found under the husk. An extract of the silk used to be officially listed in the British and American pharmacopoeias as a treatment for cystitis and kidney disorders. I have found helpful a gentle diuretic for mild cystitis made by infusing a teaspoonful of dried silk in a cup of boiling water, to be taken three times a day. However, if you have a fever, pain or blood in the urine, you should seek medical help.

‭ Figs, rhubarb and prunes

FIGS

The fig (Ficus carica) is a botanical oddity.
The many flowers form inside the familiar
pear-shaped 'fruit', and never see the light of day.
Tiny pollinating wasps crawl in through a minute aperture
and fertilise the flowers, which then develop into the seeds
that we find in a ripe fig. Originating in western Asia, the
fig soon spread and is now cultivated worldwide. There
are other related species growing elsewhere and many are
used medicinally. For example Ficus salomonensis, endemic
to the Solomon Islands, is traditionally used there to treat
constipation, just as our familiar figs are.

The ancient Egyptians valued figs for food and medicine,
as did the early Greeks, and figs are mentioned frequently
in the Bible. Being almost 50 per cent dextrose, they are
unsurprisingly popular – whether fresh or dried – and
have long formed a big part of people's staple diet in the
Mediterranean region. There was even a law passed
in classical Greece forbidding the export of the best
figs. Dried figs were found at Pompeii. The Romans
grew twenty-nine different varieties, and may have
introduced figs to Britain.

As well as their nutritive value, figs were used
medicinally. King Hezekiah's boils were treated with
figs 2,700 years ago (Isaiah 38:21), but their principal
medicinal use has always been as a gentle laxative. A
combination of high fruit sugars and fibre does the

trick. There are many ancient texts giving recipes for laxative preparations including figs, and in 1931 Syrup of Figs was still listed in the British Pharmacopoeia. A gentle version suitable for children contained figs alone; but there was a stronger version, which also included extracts of rhubarb, senna and cascara. It sounds alarming.

RHUBÁRB

My grandmother always had a bottle of Syrup of Figs in the cupboard, and as a youngster I often heard people refer to rhubarb and prunes as fruit that would also 'keep you regular'. Stewed rhubarb and custard was a favourite pudding, and rhubarb crumble was even better. Our familiar garden rhubarb is a hybrid of two Chinese species. Chinese herbal legends from 2700 BCE describe the roots of two rhubarb species as a laxative. Roots were traded commercially and eventually arrived in Europe. In his 1578 *The Garden of Health*, William Langham wrote: 'the root is good against the windiness, wambling, and weakness of the stomach' and many other afflictions, too.

The hybrid grown for the culinary use of its stems arrived in Europe in the eighteenth century. Rhubarb root should only be used under medical supervision, as it can cause problems for people with arthritis or kidney disease, and in pregnancy. Some people find that eating rhubarb stems exacerbates their arthritis, too. Rhubarb leaves, rich in oxalic acid, are potentially toxic, but the stems contain less acid – though they are still great for cleaning brass.

Prunes, the dried plums so useful as fruit in winter, also contain high levels of fructose and fibre, and are well known as a gentle laxative. Sugars are concentrated in the drying process, so dried fruit should be avoided by people with diabetes. Plums have been dried for winter use since at least Roman times, and today the very best ones come from Agen near Bordeaux, France. I had been brought up on tinned prunes, and later I used dried ones that I could soak myself – and they were pleasant enough. But it wasn't until I visited Bordeaux that I realised how truly delicious prunes can be.

◌ The garlic family

Onions and garlic belong to a large genus of plants, about seven hundred species around the world, many of which have always been valued for their flavour and medicinal properties. Some species have been cultivated for such a long time that their origins are now lost and they are no longer found in the wild.

Early texts from China, Egypt, Babylon and India all sing the praises of these plants as both food and medicine. In ancient Greece, Theophrastus wrote in detail about the cultivation of different types of onion and garlic. In the Old Testament, the Children of Israel, liberated from Egypt, complained: 'We remember the fish, which we did eat in Egypt freely; and the cucumbers, and the melons, and the leeks, and the onions, and the garlic' (Numbers 11:5). Manna from Heaven just wasn't interesting enough, apparently. In ancient Egypt, onions were used in mummification, placed inside the body, perhaps to deter snakes. Garlic was also found in many tombs, including that of Tutankhamun, and Pliny reported a belief that the very smell of garlic repelled snakes and scorpions.

ONIONS

Milk in which onions had been simmered was, within living memory, considered a suitable food for invalids, with or without 'sops' (cubes of bread). Like other members of the same genus, onions have a long-standing reputation for helping intestinal conditions, as well as respiratory disorders. Onions baked until soft and cut in half were noted in a 1980s Women's Institute recipe book as a traditional poultice to draw boils and 'gatherings'. Onion juice, used in classical times for ear infections, is in fact antibiotic, and the folk belief still persists that onions absorb both evil and infection.

LEEKS

There is a ninth-century Coptic text which, alarmingly, advocates a combination of leeks and fresh urine as an eyewash for poor night-vision. Coptic physicians also used dried leeks mixed with kohl and honey to treat genital warts.

GARLIC

The strongest member of the genus, both in flavour and
medicinal benefit, is garlic (*Allium sativum*). The genus name,
Allium, means garlic in Latin. The smell is diffusible: in
1897, a researcher reported that 'even when applied to the
soles of the feet its odour is exhaled by the lungs'. Dried
garlic pills are available for those who dislike the taste, and
'garlic breath' can be reduced temporarily by eating lots of
parsley.

Garlic has been shown to reduce blood pressure, blood-
sugar and cholesterol levels, and it is both antibiotic and
antiseptic. High-concentration garlic extract can interact
with blood-thinning medication, but garlic in the diet
is generally safe. In the Middle Ages, people used it as a
prophylactic against the plague, which swept across Europe
at periodic intervals. Physicians recognised its healing
properties a long time ago: Dioscorides prescribed garlic
for all respiratory and intestinal disorders occurring among
the soldiers in his care. In the early twentieth century,
doctors working in Dublin and New York published research
attesting to the effectiveness of garlic in the treatment of
tuberculosis and whooping cough, both major causes of
death at the time. In the middle of the twentieth century,
researchers found that garlic had a beneficial
effect on the gut flora: it destroyed 'bad bacteria'
while allowing 'good bacteria' to flourish,
confirming that ancient physicians were
right to suggest garlic for intestinal
disorders.

Garlic also had a reputation as a treatment for skin disorders and wound healing, though it could raise blisters, and so had to be applied with care. In the Second World War, the British government bought vast quantities of garlic to treat soldiers' wounds: not one case of septic poisoning was reported among those treated with garlic. Russian military doctors reported similar findings. Some have found garlic helpful in relieving painful rheumatic joints, though I would not advise rubbing raw garlic onto the skin, as directed by some early writers. Instead, I would follow the ancient Indian advice of massaging with oil in which garlic has been fried.

Many of the world's wild allium species are edible too, but do consult a good identification guide when foraging for them in the woods. The onion smell is a positive clue. But beware of introducing wild allium species into your garden, as some of them can be very invasive.

A soothing cough mixture

When afflicted with a cough, I slice an onion into a bowl, pour runny honey over it, cover and leave it overnight. In the morning, I pour off the liquor – a soothing linctus, which keeps for several days in the fridge. I take a teaspoonful of this three or four times a day. Both onion juice and honey have antiseptic and expectorant properties. And it tastes better than you might expect!

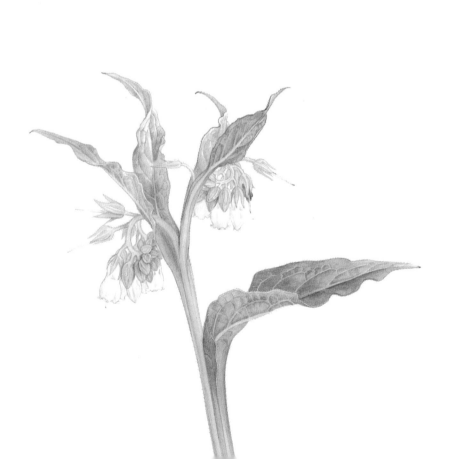

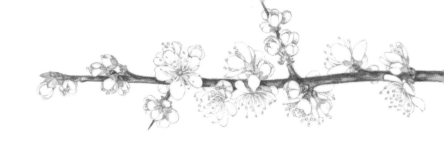

Spring

When the season begins to smile

THEOPHRASTUS (371–c.287 BCE),
Enquiry into Plants

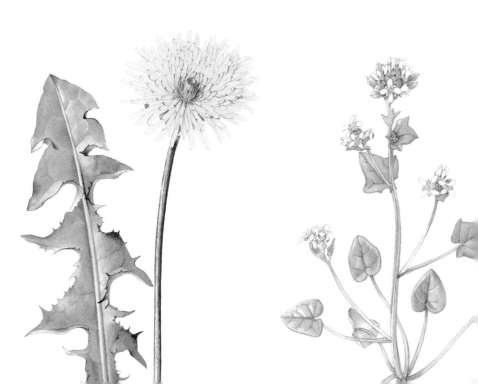

A fter the cold, dark days of winter, spring is a welcome relief to us – and must have been even more so to our forebears. It is a time for looking forward, for planting and pruning to ensure an abundant harvest to come, both for the table and for the medicine cabinet.

∾ Celandines

The name 'celandine' is applied to two totally unrelated plants with nothing in common botanically, but both having yellow flowers. Both are native to Europe and western Asia and are naturalised in North America. The first to bloom, on roadsides and hedge banks, is lesser celandine, with its starry flowers against slightly glossy, dark-green leaves. Unusually among British wildflowers, it has glossy petals, too, like its close relatives, the buttercups. Until very recently it was classified with the buttercups as a *Ranunculus*, but is now called *Ficaria verna*. *Ficaria* is a medieval name derived from *ficus*, the Latin for 'fig', because its knobbly root-tubers look a bit like tiny white figs. 'Fig' was also a slang term for piles (haemorrhoids), so the plant was also called 'figwort' or 'pilewort', and was made into an ointment for piles. Dr John Hill in 1756 said the roots were 'cooling and softening … an excellent remedy in the pain of the piles'. They would also help with 'scrophulous tumours', he said. Lesser celandine was sometimes taken internally as an infusion; but neither external nor internal treatment is used today. If you are tempted to introduce lesser celandine into your garden, be aware that it will spread everywhere.

Lesser and greater celandine illustrate the complicated web of common names, classical allusions and folk tales that entangle our familiar plants. 'Celandine' is an anglicisation of *chelidon*, the Greek name for the swallow. Greater celandine goes by the scientific name *Chelidonium majus*, and its alternative common name is 'swallow-wort'. Some said this was because it flowered at about the time that swallows reappeared and finished flowering when they left; but there grew up a story that mother swallows bathed their blind nestlings' eyes with its juice to help them see.

This story was repeated down the ages and seemed to suggest that greater celandine would be a suitable treatment for eye problems. Many writers from Aristotle onwards scoffed at the story – everyone knew that nestlings would open their eyes and see without any interventions – but it did not prevent them from recommending the herb in optical preparations. The tenth-century *Leechbook of Bald* lists many eye treatments, the majority of them including greater celandine. One recipe is copied directly from Dioscorides, some 850 years before. Following in the same footsteps, Gerard said in 1597: 'The juice of the herb … cleans and consumes away slimy things that cleave about the ball of the eye, and hinder the sight, and especially being boiled with honey in a brazen vessel, as Dioscorides teaches.' I'm all for clearing away 'slimy things', but the orange sap of greater celandine is dangerously corrosive. When heated gently it was said to become less irritant and more effective, especially when mixed with bactericidal honey, but please don't try it.

Greater celandine's other virtue, attested to by a historical and widespread folk tradition, is its reputation for healing warts. Its sap can severely irritate healthy skin, so you had to be careful to apply it only to the wart itself. Greater celandine is most often found growing wild near habitation, and historically it was grown for its medicinal value, as well as for its attractive glaucous foliage and small, butter-yellow flowers in summer. It seeds freely, but all parts of it are poisonous.

But what does *lesser* celandine have to do with swallows? It flowers before they arrive and is over well before they depart. Towards the end of the eighteenth century, Gilbert White recorded its peak flowering at Selborne in Hampshire beginning around 21 February, and similar dates have been recorded ever since. Perhaps, as Richard Mabey surmises, it was, like the swallow, a herald of a kinder season. Which is why many people love it – its cheerful yellow stars are so heartening after a dark winter. It was Wordsworth's favourite flower: he wrote no fewer than three poems about it and noted how its flowers open in the sun, reminding us that spring is on its way.

❧ Violets

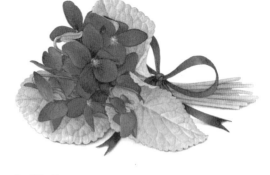

'Violet' is a name that
in the past was given
to several different
sweet-smelling plants,
including wallflowers and gillyflowers,
while the plants we today know as violets were called 'March
violets'. We have several native violet species in Europe, and
there are many more around the world. In Britain, the best
known is the sweet violet (*Viola odorata*). It is the earliest to
flower and is the one most used in medicine. It is the only
one of our native species with a scent. The purple, nodding
flowers are not conspicuous, but their alluring perfume is
striking. Often, as poet John Clare wrote, 'they smell before
they're seen'. Natural variation in one of our scent receptors
means that some people are unable to detect the fragrance,
while for others it appears to come and go.

People have always delighted in violet flowers, making
them into attractive, fragrant garlands or posies which were
considered beneficial, too. The Romans wore chaplets of
violets to ward off drunkenness and to relieve hangovers
and headaches. Medieval households added the fresh flowers
to their strewing herbs, scattered them in salads, and made
breath-freshening cachous from them.

Infusions of violet leaves and flowers have been popular
since classical times in Europe to treat headaches and for
coughs. They do contain methyl salicylate, related to aspirin,
which could explain their enduring popularity. Russian
traditional folk medicine recommended a decoction of violet

flowers to treat tonsillitis, while infusions and poultices were thought to help in certain types of cancer. In the 1930s, British writer Mrs Grieve reported that extracts of sweet violet had been used successfully in the treatment of tongue and throat cancers, and recent research appears to suggest encouraging results in other cancers, too.

Syrup of Violets

Remove the calyxes from three handfuls of sweet violet flowers. Boil about 150ml (¼ pint) of water in a small pan.

Allow to cool slightly, then add the flowers, stir and cover.

Allow to stand for 24 hours. Strain, pressing the pulp gently.

To every cup of liquid add two cups of white sugar.

In a bain-marie (or a bowl set over a pan of simmering water) gently warm the syrup, stirring until the sugar is dissolved.

In her 1670 cookery book, Hannah Woolley recommended adding a drop or two of lemon juice to keep the syrup a good, transparent purple. Poured into sterilised bottles or jars, this will keep for six months or more in the fridge.

I dilute a teaspoonful in a cup of warm water for a cold or a sore throat, or use it in baking or cocktails. It does make a sensational icing to drizzle over cakes.

The lovely fragrance is lost when the flowers are dried, but it transfers easily to liquid preparations. Syrup of Violets was listed in the British Pharmacopoeia as late as the 1930s as a gentle laxative for young children, but is now marketed to add to cocktails and ice cream. Sweet violet grows well in my shady garden, so I have no need to raid the hedge-banks and woods to make violet syrup.

❧ Coltsfoot (colt's-foot)

As a child, I always thought there was something mysterious about coltsfoot (*Tussilago farfara*). On a damp bank near the river where my friends and I used to play, scaly spikes would appear in the early spring, each topped with a yellow, daisy-like flower. Not until after the flower spikes had withered away would the big, heart-shaped, jagged-edged leaves appear. I didn't know it at the time, but one of its country names is 'son before the father' for that very reason. The two stages of its growth are so very different that several of the early printed herbals show two separate illustrations to aid identification at different times of the year.

Coltsfoot is so called because the shape of its leaves resembles a hoof print, though in some areas it is called after different hoofed animals: 'bull-foot', 'horse-hoof' and so on. The undersides of the leaves are covered with a white fluff which, dried and mixed with saltpetre, made a useful tinder. Coltsfoot's scientific name *Tussilago* comes from the Latin *tussis*, meaning 'cough', an indication of its main medicinal virtue. Since very early times, coltsfoot has been used to treat all kinds of coughs and bronchial disorders. In the sixteenth century, a decoction or a syrup made from the fresh leaves and roots was suggested as an excellent cough remedy. I dimly remember as a child hearing about 'coltsfoot candy' or 'coltsfoot rock' being given as a cough remedy. It was made from sugar and coltsfoot roots. Culpeper says: 'The root is small and white, spreading much under ground, so that where it takes it will hardly be driven away again, if any little piece be abiding therein; and from thence spring fresh leaves.' So it was not an ideal plant for the herb garden.

Several historical authors also recommended smoking dried coltsfoot leaves to treat coughs – definitely not a treatment promoted today. Herb-gatherers would look for coltsfoot flowers and mark the spot to return to later in the year. This was to avoid confusing coltsfoot leaves with the similar-looking leaves of butterbur (*Petasites* spp), which were seldom used medicinally but were indeed handy for wrapping butter. Herbal tobacco, popular throughout the twentieth century, was largely composed of coltsfoot and had a reputation as a healthy alternative to tobacco.

Sir John Clerk, who was plainly very concerned with his own health, experimented by mixing coltsfoot with his regular tobacco in equal measure. He wrote in 1749 that after a year's trial he had less cough than formerly, despite being seventy-two years old. He said he had read about this in Pliny's *Natural History*, but there are many records of less-literate people employing the same treatment. Pliny did indeed advocate treating an obstinate cough with smoke

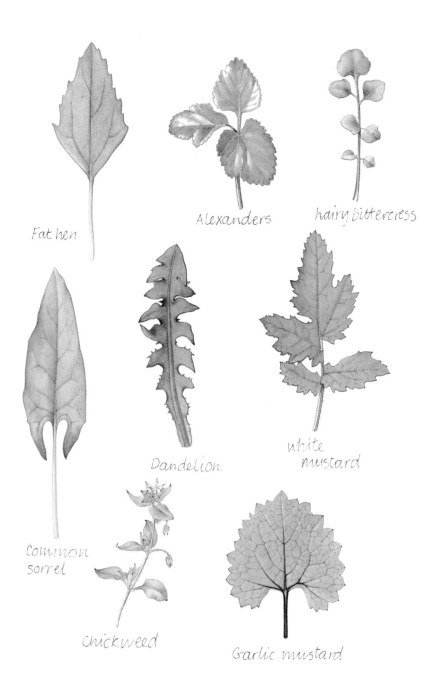

Fat hen

Alexanders

hairy bittercress

Dandelion

white
mustard

Common
sorrel

Chickweed

Garlic mustard

from dried coltsfoot leaves, preferably burning on cypress charcoal and inhaled through a reed. A sip of wine was to be taken between each inhalation. It sounds uncomfortably like some student parties I recall.

⌀ Sorrels, docks and other spring greens

In the days before polytunnels and a global food industry that thinks nothing of jetting produce around the world, most people ate whatever was in season. The wealthy had hothouses and the staff to work in them, but the majority of people were used to what the journalist Katharine Whitehorn called 'the steady march of the seasons across the dinner table'. Winter fare could be rather dull, with fewer fruits and vegetables, plus whatever had been dried, pickled or preserved during more abundant months. So when the first green weeds began to show in spring, they were a welcome change.

CHICKWEED

Regarded as an unwanted weed in summer, chickweed (*Stellaria media*) is among the earliest spring greens – in mild areas it can even persist through the winter. Early in the year it is perhaps more welcome, and not just for feeding poultry and cage birds. As well as supplying much-needed vitamin C, it also provided poultices and ointments for ulcers and inflamed skin. The leaves are too small to strip individually, so the whole plant was used.

BITTERCRESS

Bittercress (*Cardamine hirsuta*) can also be found growing
in winter and early spring, and tastes better than its name
implies. I often see it growing in my plant tubs and put a few
of its tangy leaves into winter salads, along with any young
dandelion and garlic-mustard leaves I can find.

COMMON SORREL

As the weather improves and the days lengthen, so the choice
also improves. Common sorrel (*Rumex acetosa*) has been eaten
and used in medicine since ancient times. Its leaves, shaped
like an arrow-head, have a sharp, slightly lemony flavour.
It makes a good sauce (more popular in France than it is in
Britain), which goes well with rich meat. In 1670, Hannah
Woolley gave recipes for sauces made with the closely
related French sorrel, which, she said, were good with meat
or served on their own for 'a sick body' to eat. Nineteenth-
century farmworkers chewed sorrel leaves to quench their
thirst, and herbalists said that the roots were good for the
heart, while the leaves – eaten raw in a salad – were excellent
for the blood. However, sorrel contains oxalic acid, too much
of which can cause kidney stones.

WOOD SORREL

The unrelated native wood sorrel (*Oxalis acetosella*), with
its light-green trifoliate leaves and dainty white nodding
flowers, also had a reputation for quenching thirst. It was

made into a sauce ideal with fish, and in medieval England was cultivated especially for this purpose. It, too, contains vitamin C and oxalic acid. It was also called 'allelujah', and in his herbal, published in 1568, William Turner explained this was 'because it appears about Easter when allelujah is sung again [after Lent]'. This name was common in France and Italy, too. Wood sorrel shared the detoxifying, tonic reputation ascribed to many of the 'bitter herbs' eaten at this time of year. Bitter herbs were considered appropriate for both body and soul during the Lenten fast. And even today there is still the lingering suspicion that if something tastes bitter it must be doing you good.

SCURVY GRASS

One of the most bitter-tasting was scurvy grass, named because it was a recognised treatment for scurvy, caused by vitamin C deficiency. Danish scurvy grass (Cochlearia danica) is, despite its name, a pan-European native that is usually coastal, but now flourishes along roads that are salted in winter. Its salty bitterness can be reduced by soaking it in fresh water. It was famously eaten by sailors, and spread to the east coast of America, providing a convenient supply for the return voyage. A 1688 English household book gives a complicated, ale-based scurvy treatment that includes scurvy grass, so lack of vitamin C evidently affected the landlocked, too.

DOCKS

Many docks – called 'dockens' in the north of England and in Scotland – were also eaten and were thought to cleanse the system. American dock species were considered good blood cleansers, too. In Britain, broad-leaved dock (*Rumex obtusifolius*) was known as butter-dock, as its leaves were used to wrap butter. This and curled dock (*Rumex crispa*) taste especially bitter. Rather surprisingly, when on a botanical trip to Armenia, I saw women collecting curled dock to dry for winter stores. Long, plaited ropes of it were sold in the markets and you just cut off a length to add to your winter stew. Perhaps they had a secret way of lessening the bitterness.

A dock known as 'monk's rhubarb' was cultivated in ancient Britain, and patience dock was introduced in 1573 to grow for the table, though Culpeper remarked that our native 'bloodwort' (red-veined or wood dock, *Rumex sanguineus*) was 'as wholesome a pot-herb as any that grows in a garden'; it also strengthened the liver and cleaned the blood. Country folk made dock leaves into poultices for wounds and rheumatism. However, the best-known therapeutic use of dock is rubbing a leaf onto nettle stings. People have been doing this for a very long time: Chaucer quotes a well-established rhyme about it in his poem *Troilus and Criseyde*, written in the mid-1380s.

Dock and bistort (*Persicaria* spp) were two of the ingredients in 'herb pudding' or 'Easter ledge pudding' made in the north of England. The leaves were chopped, mixed with nettles, parsley, barley, oatmeal, butter and egg, and steamed in a cloth. These spring greens were all believed to be a beneficial tonic, and today adding a few leaves to a salad, soup or stew is fun as well, providing you are certain you have identified them correctly. An old proverb from the Channel Islands says: 'Eat leeks with sorrel in March, cresses in April, and ramsons in May, and all the year after physicians may go play.'

ꙮ Mahonia

Many gardeners grow mahonia bushes for their evergreen leaves and sweet-scented yellow flowers in early spring. Mahonias originate in Asia and North America, but are now grown everywhere with a temperate climate, and are sometimes planted in British woods as pheasant cover. I especially love the spiky leaflets turning crimson as they age, and the bunches of berries that look like miniature grapes. These berries gave the plant its common name of 'Oregon grape' and were used by the Ditidaht and Nlaka'pamux nations in Canada as a laxative. Asian *Mahonia* species have been used in traditional Chinese medicine for digestive and skin disorders, just as the shorter, more

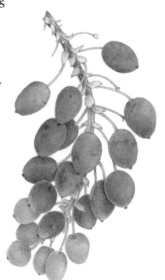

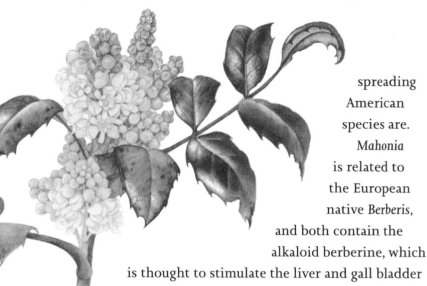

spreading
American
species are.
Mahonia
is related to
the European
native *Berberis*,
and both contain the
alkaloid berberine, which
is thought to stimulate the liver and gall bladder
and to cleanse the blood of toxins. However,
berberine should never be used without first
consulting your doctor or healthcare provider and should
always be avoided in pregnancy and during lactation, as it
may harm the foetus or the new-born child. Mahonia has
a reputation for lowering blood pressure and blood sugar
and for thinning the blood. However, people already on
medication for such conditions or for diabetes should
seek medical advice before taking mahonia,
as the berberine it contains could interact
dangerously with their medication.

The Squaxin of North America, among
many other groups, made decoctions
of mahonia roots or bark as a blood-
purifying tonic, and more recently
mahonia has been used to treat
skin conditions such as psoriasis
and eczema. Applying a poultice or
gel can reduce pain and redness of
the skin, but, again, you should take

medical advice before using it if you are pregnant or nursing. *Mahonia aquifolium* and *Mahonia* (or *Berberis*) *repens* were the species used most often, but some tribes made remedies for sore eyes and even tuberculosis from whatever species they found locally. There are records that the Paiute gave the roots of *Mahonia repens* 'to thicken the blood of haemophilic persons', though I could find no reports of how successful this was.

○ Dandelions

The name dandelion is said to be a corruption of the French *dent-de-lion*, 'lion's tooth', and in medieval Latin it was *dens leonis*, which means the same thing. In his 1548 *The Names of Herbes*, William Turner called it *dan de lyon* and said 'it groweth everywhere'. Perhaps the name was inspired by the jagged leaves which, if you try hard enough, could be thought to resemble jaws full of savage teeth. When I first started learning scientific names, the dandelion was *Taraxacum officinale*, the second part suggesting that this was an 'official' medicinal plant. However, recent research suggests that the species is, in fact, a large group of closely related micro-species. Well over two hundred micro-species are recognised in the British Isles alone, forty of them endemic – i.e. not found anywhere else. This is not the place to explore the botanical intricacies of the *Taraxacum* 'aggregation': we all know a dandelion when we see one. Unlike yellow-flowered lookalikes, the dandelion has an unbranched hollow stem, all its leaves in a basal rosette and all parts of it are hairless.

Unwelcome in most gardens, it is easy to find in fields, on road verges and waste ground everywhere in the northern hemisphere.

Although a very common plant, it has inspired poetry by Shakespeare, Keats and Walt Whitman, among others; and it figures in work by artists from Albrecht Dürer to Andy Goldsworthy. Its golden-yellow flowers, 'shining like guineas', are hard to ignore and are followed by what Gerard called 'a round, downy blowball that is carried away by the wind'. We all blew on 'dandelion clocks' as children. The remaining bald, tonsure-like receptacle, surrounded by its turned-down bracts, gave it the name of 'priest's crown'. But it is the ubiquitous common names of 'wet-the-bed' and 'piss-a-bed' that hint at its medicinal qualities. The leaves are a powerful diuretic, helpful in relieving kidney problems, and the roots stimulate the liver and gall bladder. The taraxacin in the whole plant encourages the production of bile, which helps the digestive process.

Dandelion leaves have been employed as a diuretic for at least 2,000 years in Chinese and Ayurvedic medicine, as well as in the western tradition. They are eaten in salads, too, and were included in a 1525 list of 'Herbs necessary for a Garden'. In the days before modern lettuce varieties, wealthier families would grow dandelions in a greenhouse for winter salads. The leaves are rather bitter unless picked when young, or blanched by growing them under an upturned pot. They contain vitamins A, B, C and D, as well as significant amounts of iron and potassium, minerals which are often lost when using other diuretics.

Decoctions of the roots have been recommended for liver complaints and as a blood-cleansing tonic in printed herbals and household notebooks alike for many centuries. The roots are best dug in November, but do not keep well when dried, and so need to be replaced annually. Roasted, ground roots were even used as an additive to, or substitute for, coffee when it was hard to get in Britain during the Second World War.

The flowers can be added to salads, but are best known for making a delicate wine. Tradition had it that the best wine was made from flowers collected on St George's Day, 23 April (or 12 April by the old calendar). My mother used to make it in a huge stoneware vat, with the yeast spread onto a piece of toast floating on top. Dandelion beer was a popular drink, especially among workers in steel works or potteries, who were in danger of dehydration from the furnaces and kilns. And 'dandelion and burdock' was a drink well known in my childhood, made from the roots, plus ginger, sugar and lemon juice. It was considered an excellent tonic and tasted delicious.

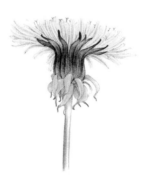

∾ Cowslips

Cowslips (Primula veris)
and primroses (Primula
vulgaris) both belong to the
Primula genus, and hybridise to produce
the false oxlip, the main parent of our
popular garden polyanthus. All members
of the genus hybridise prolifically, often
producing a 'hybrid swarm' of plants of
varying shapes, sizes and colours.
Cowslips are native to
Europe and western Asia.
The word 'Primula' is a
diminutive of the Latin
primus, meaning 'first', and
in medieval times the name
Primula veris was applied to many
spring wildflowers, especially the
daisy. Some early herbal writers
instead called the cowslip Radix arthritica, because
its roots were used to relieve the pain of arthritis. They do in
fact contain salicylates which may have helped, though their
main virtue was in treating whooping cough and bronchitis.
Primrose roots were also used; but, as some writers reported,
they could cause violent vomiting.

Old herbals sometimes gave cowslip the name Paralysis
vulgaris, echoing the country name 'palsy-wort' and hinting
at another medicinal use. Since antiquity, healers have
administered the flowers and leaves to relieve palsy (paralysis

and tremor). A fifteenth-century manuscript recommended cowslip and lavender flowers boiled in ale 'for trembling hand and hands asleep'. Later writers prescribed a syrup or conserve of cowslip flowers for the same disorders. Surviving private household books, as well as printed herbals, give recipes for delicious and delicate cowslip wine, used – in medicinal doses, of course – to treat insomnia and nervous tension. In 1756, John Hill wrote that a syrup or conserve of cowslip flowers had 'a gently narcotic quality' and would 'mitigate pain, promote perspiration, and dispose gently to sleep'. Country people drank cowslip flower tea to relieve a headache, and in 1860 'paigle' tea was noted as a children's teatime treat.

Cowslips have attracted a good deal of folklore and have acquired many country names, such as paigles or St Peter's keys, from the flowers nodding in a bunch at the top of the stem. 'Cowslip' is a polite version of 'cowslop' (cow-pat), as cowslips were thought to grow best in cattle pastures. People thought the flowers' sweet fragrance came from the orange spots inside. In A Midsummer Night's Dream, one of the fairies explains:

> In their gold coats spots you see,
> Those be rubies, fairy favours,
> In those freckles live their savours.

Perhaps it was their sweet scent that led to their use in cosmetic preparations. Cowslip ointment has long been applied for sunburn, spots and to soften the skin. In the mid-sixteenth century, William Turner wrote that some women washed their faces with a distillation of cowslip flowers 'to drive wrinkles away and to make them fair in the eyes of the world rather than in the eyes of God, Whom they are not afraid to offend'. Rather harsh, I feel.

Cowslips were once very common, but with so much old grassland having been ploughed up and with the increased use of pesticides, there has been a catastrophic decline since the 1950s. I love driving along a Dorset road which skirts a nature reserve, whose hillsides are yellow with cowslips in late April. That is now a very rare sight. Fortunately, in recent decades management practices have changed, and cowslips are creeping back to roadsides and field edges, though they are still too uncommon to pick in the numbers we used to as children. Picking cowslips for wine or tea is no longer sustainable, unless you grow your own. They can be grown in gardens – and have been since at least the Middle Ages – if you have an alkaline soil and plenty of sunshine. They should be divided every other year and they flower noticeably better after sub-zero winter temperatures.

✍ Stinging nettles

Our ancestors ate nettles (Urtica dioica) as a spring vegetable, and many of us still do. In February 1661, Samuel Pepys wrote in his diary that he had tried 'nettle porridge' and had enjoyed it. A dish made with oatmeal, nettles and sometimes other ingredients, such as leeks and broccoli, was well known in the north of England and in Scotland as 'nettle pudding'. The stings disappear with cooking or drying. The tops of young shoots, gathered in March, can be steamed like spinach, puréed or added to soups.

A nineteenth-century collection of traditional Scottish rhymes includes this suggestion to substitute nettles for 'lang kail' (a kind of cabbage leaf):

> Gin ye be for lang kail
> Cou' the nettle, stoo the nettle,
> Gin ye be for lang kail
> Cou' the nettle early.

The many old rhymes about gathering nettles in March are not just superstition: as the plants mature and flower, so the leaves become coarse and unpalatable, and even slightly toxic. Eaten young, they are a good source of vitamins A and C and iron. I often get my thick gardening gloves on and collect spring nettle tops to dry for nettle tea. Old books recommend cutting nettles back in high summer to get a second flush of young growth, but several of our best-known butterfly species lay their eggs on nettle leaves, so I search the plants carefully before cutting.

Stinging nettles are native to Europe, but have spread to temperate regions everywhere. English traveller and writer John Josselyn recorded them growing wild in New England as early as 1672. Nettles were encouraged, as they were so useful. A decoction in salty water provides a vegetable rennet to curdle milk for cheese. A decoction of leaves makes a good hair conditioner and, according to Pliny, prevents hair loss. Nettles flourish in nitrogen-rich soil, especially near human habitation, and an isolated patch of nettles can indicate where a settlement once stood even centuries before.

Nettles had other uses, too: the fibres have been made into cloth since at least the Bronze Age. In Germany during the First World War, some military clothing contained up to 85 per cent nettle fibre. Some Himalayan and Chinese species of nettle are made into soft, silky luxury cloth. Nettles also give yellow or green dyes, and during the Second World War the County Herb Committees in Britain oversaw the collection of nettles for dyeing camouflage fabric.

Nettles were, like many spring plants, thought to cleanse the blood. Nettle tea and nettle beer have a long-standing reputation as tonics, and as treatments for rheumatism and arthritis. A more brutal treatment was 'urtication', which involved beating or rubbing inflamed painful joints with fresh nettles. Urtication has a long history in European folk medicine, stretching back to the Romans. Some scientific studies suggest that nettles may help with rheumatism and arthritis through both internal and external treatment. I would happily recommend nettle tea, but draw the line at urtication.

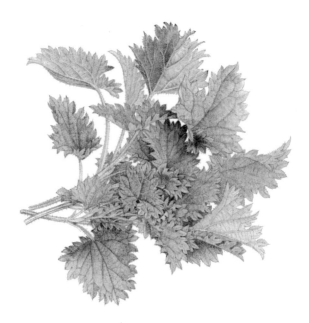

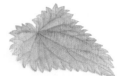

Nettle and lemon balm tea
(adapted from an old Devonshire recipe)

Put a small handful of young nettle tops and a large handful of fresh lemon balm leaves into a jug. Add a few cloves, and lemon juice and honey to taste.

Pour on 600ml (1 pint) of boiling water, cover and allow to stand for an hour, then strain.

I take a warmed cupful at night for a cold.

It will keep for a day or two in the fridge, but you could freeze it for future use. I find it a refreshing cold summer drink, too.

You can make it with dried nettle leaves, but the balm needs to be fresh.

∾ Plantains

Even the commonest native plants may have medicinal virtue. Pollen analysis shows that plantains – Plantago species, not the tropical foodplant of the same name – increased dramatically with Neolithic forest clearance for agriculture, so it has been common in Europe for a very long time. Theophrastus referred to it as a flower without petals, though the flowers, packed into a crowded inflorescence, do in fact have tiny, cream-coloured petals flattened against the flowerhead. The hard, round heads of ribwort plantain have featured in children's games since remote antiquity: as a child, I had no idea of the ancient heritage of whacking my friend's 'soldier' with one of my own. In some areas this game is called 'kemps', probably from the Anglo-Saxon word *cempa*, meaning 'soldier'.

There are many different plantain species, but by far the commonest British natives are common or broad-leaved plantain (*Plantago major*), which grows on disturbed ground, and ribwort plantain (*Plantago lanceolata*), which is common in meadows and grassland. Both are now found all over the world. In seventeenth-century New England, John Josselyn reported that Native Americans had named common plantain 'English man's foot', as it sprang up wherever the settlers went 'as though produced by their treading'. The Cherokee, among others, used its leaves to treat insect bites, stings, blisters and burns. I have applied plantain leaves to relieve insect bites and stings, and have even seen them calm horse-fly bites if applied straightaway. I simply pick a clean leaf, mash it up a little to get the juices flowing, and rub it on the afflicted part.

Common plantain was certainly popular in England both medicinally and as food, hence its Old English name of 'waybread'. The leaves were cooked or added to salads, and the nutty-tasting seeds are a good source of protein. I grow ribwort plantain in my garden to treat insect bites. It seeds freely, but is easy enough to weed out where it isn't wanted. I leave plenty of seeds for the birds, who love them. People used to collect bunches of seeding plantain for their cage birds to eat. The southern European Plantago psyllium (or Plantago indica) has very mucilaginous seeds, which are used, like flax seed, as a gentle bulk laxative.

Both the common plantains were credited with healing all manner of complaints. Dioscorides prescribed them for wounds, ulcers and sores, and the Lacnunga, a tenth-century collection of herbal remedies, listed plantain among the nine sacred herbs. In 1390, poet John Gower wrote: '... and of Plantain he has his herb sovereign'. It is mentioned as a healing herb in several of Shakespeare's plays, so it was plainly well known to his audience. Herbal writers recommended it as good for the bowels, head, eyes, ears and skin, for stopping bleeding and 'all manner of fluxes', and to relieve pain, especially toothache. Gerard reported that there were many more outlandish and superstitious claims for its powers, but declined to list such 'ridiculous toys'. Chemical analysis shows that plantains do contain several vitamins, tannins, salicylic acid (related to aspirin), glycosides and mucilage, so they may well have had some beneficial effects.

❧ Milkwort

On a botanical holiday in eastern Europe, I spotted a relative of our tiny milkworts (Polygala spp), and remarked to my neighbour that these flowers were once thought to

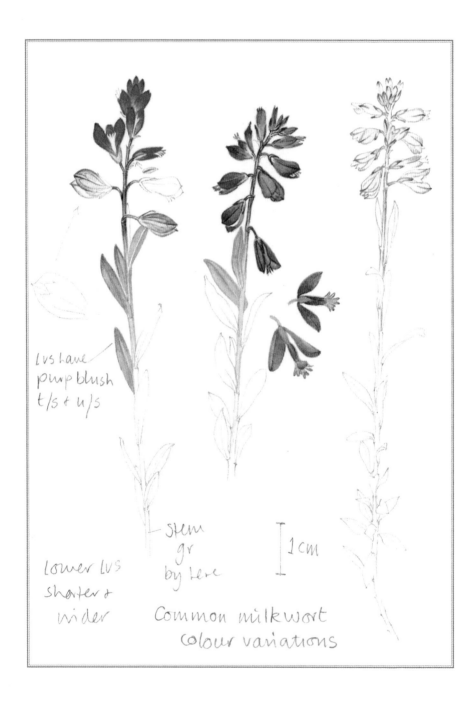

lvs have
purp blush
t/s + u/s

Lower lvs
shorter +
wider

stem
gr
by here

1cm

Common milkwort
Colour variations

promote milk in nursing mothers. He pulled a face and dismissed the idea out of hand. It turned out that he was a medical doctor who considered all herbal treatments to be superstitious nonsense. I think if I was a medieval mother without modern medical help, I would have tried anything to save my baby from starving. However, I suspect that milkwort wasn't a very effective treatment – it is not mentioned at all in many herbals, and there are few records in the oral tradition either. It was described by Dioscorides and other ancient writers, but their term *polygalon* (which does mean 'much milk') may refer to livestock browsing on pastures where milkwort grew, rather than to human nursing mothers. And of course, they might have meant a different plant altogether.

Native milkworts grow in short grass in various habitats across much of Europe, and there are bigger, shrubby species native to other parts of the world. Several North American species were used as remedies – by the Sioux for earache, the Seminole for heart trouble, the Blackfoot and many others for pulmonary complaints, for example – but I can find no mention of American milkworts promoting breast milk.

Gerard describes a milkwort flower beautifully: 'of a blue colour, fashioned like a little bird, with wings, tail, and body easy to be discerned by them that do observe the same'. This bird-like form is even easier to see in some of the larger, shrubby species now grown in gardens. Gerard remarks upon the confusion between British milkworts and similar plants, and claims that our different species of milkwort can be distinguished by the colour of their flowers. Having been tasked with illustrating all the British native milkworts for a field guide, I doubt his assertion: each of our species can have flowers that vary from dark to very pale blue – or, in the case of our two commonest, pink or white as well. I think these are plants to admire, rather than to use.

∾ Milkweed

The name 'milkwort' is often confused with 'milkweed', members of the genus *Asclepias*, named after the Greek god of healing, and in a totally different family of plants. They are 2 or 3 feet tall, with sprays of small pink, orange or yellow flowers. Another name is 'silkweed', because of the silky fluff that encloses the seeds. Most members of the genus are native to the Americas, the West Indies or South Africa, and most are poisonous. However, like some other poisonous plants, they have been taken as medicine, with an appropriately small dose of a specific part.

The Navajo, among many others, are recorded as using *Asclepias* species for a variety of complaints, especially respiratory disorders. The Miwok and Cherokee applied the milky sap (which gives the plants their name) to cure warts. Pink-flowered swamp milkweed (*Asclepias incarnata*) was taken by the Iroquois and Meskwaki as a diuretic, which Mrs Grieve reported was 'quick and certain'; others used it for dysentery, asthma and worms.

Another species, *Asclepias tuberosa*, is known as 'pleurisy root'. Once listed in the official US Pharmacopoeia, it was said to relieve breathing difficulties and mitigate the pain of pleurisy. Although slightly less toxic than its relatives, it could still be powerfully emetic and purgative. Milkweeds contain cardiac glycosides, which in small doses can create confusion, but in high doses can induce seizures, arrhythmia, respiratory paralysis and even death. So definitely not recommended for home use.

It is a lovely garden plant, however, and attracts insects with its sweetly scented flowers. Driving in Hungary, I was surprised to see that *Asclepias syriaca* was often the dominant roadside flora. Apparently this is a relic of a historical initiative to kick-start a Hungarian honey industry, when fields of milkweed were planted for the bees. Unfortunately, lacking its native predators, it has become invasive.

❧ Comfrey

Well known to ancient physicians and herbalists, comfrey (*Symphytum officinale*) has always been a favourite healing herb. Dioscorides called it *Symphytum*, which derives from a Greek term meaning 'to unite', and its species name *officinale* indicates that it was on the official list of medicinal plants – it was on the list, in fact, right up to the mid-eighteenth century. In 1548, William Turner reported that it was known to herbalists as *Consolida majorem*, the greatest of the consolidating, joining herbs.

In 1694, John Pechey wrote: 'outwardly applied it stops the blood of wounds and helps to unite broken bones; whereof 'tis called bone-set'. There have been many reports down the years of folk healers using its roots to set broken bones.

Comfrey contains a great deal of mucilage (which soothes inflammation) and allantoin (which promotes cell growth and aids healing). The boiled leaves, applied as a poultice, would set hard, making a good splint. Several authors repeated the boast that it healed so well and so quickly that if you grated some fresh comfrey root into a stew, it would join the chunks of meat together.

Several species of comfrey grow wild in Europe, and plants taken to New England soon naturalised there, too. Britain's native common comfrey (Symphytum officinale) has large, slightly rough leaves – Culpeper says they will make your hands itch – and pale cream or pinkish nodding flowers in a coiled raceme, like all the borage family. Russian comfrey (Symphytum x uplandicum) was introduced to Britain in 1870 as a fodder crop, though livestock are not very keen on it. Other introduced species have hybridised, backcrossed and escaped, so there is a range of flower colours and features among the plants growing wild on roadsides and in fields. Comfrey is a popular garden plant, especially varieties with blue, purple or pure white flowers, though it can become invasive. Gardeners sometimes dig it in as a green manure.

All types of comfrey were used for medicinal purposes. Infusions and decoctions of comfrey were prescribed for internal ulcers and ruptures. Gerard recommended drinking comfrey root in ale for backache 'gotten by any violent motion, as wrestling, or overmuch use of women'. Though he also noted that the treatment could cause involuntary ejaculation. Studies have shown that taking comfrey internally can indeed affect the sex hormones. Historically, comfrey was eaten as a vegetable or in salad. I have been given comfrey soup in France and, thankfully, didn't notice any unexpected effects. In the middle of the last century, young leaves fried in batter were a popular spring delicacy in Bavaria. However, modern research has discovered that comfrey contains alkaloids which, in large doses, can cause liver damage, so it should not be taken internally. The alkaloids can be absorbed through the skin, so long-term external use or use on broken skin should be avoided, unless you are using alkaloid-free preparations.

Comfrey's safety during pregnancy and lactation, or for use on children, has not been established, so it should not be used.

However, today, prepared as creams and ointments, and used as prescribed by a health practitioner, comfrey can bring benefits. In rigorous medical tests, creams made with extracts of the root (with the dangerous alkaloid removed) confirmed comfrey's power to ease painful joints in arthritis, gout and sprains. Another study showed that a product containing an extract of Russian comfrey leaves significantly improved wound healing. So, used externally with care, and under medical supervision, comfrey can continue its healing tradition.

ᴄᴡ Bugle

As spring moves towards summer and more plants begin to flower, one of the prettiest and most valued medicinally is common bugle (*Ajuga reptans*). Related to sage, betony and the woundworts, bugle was reckoned among the 'consounds' or wound herbs known as *Consolida media*. Vernacular names such as 'sicklewort' and 'carpenter's herb' confirm its reputation, though people also used some of the same names for self-heal. In North America, the name 'bugleweed' is sometimes applied to common bugle, but also to other plants – illustrating yet again how useful scientific names can be.

In the sixteenth century, as now, bugle was common in damp, shady woods and copses, and was much planted in gardens. It appears in medieval garden lists – and no wonder, for its spires of lavender-blue flowers against its dark-green leaves are very attractive. It spreads by runners, so can make useful ground cover in shady spots. The colour of the leaves is hard to describe: one writer called it 'a black herb', while another described the leaves as brown. In fact, a fourteenth-century name for it was *wodebroun*, 'wood-brown'. Having painted it many times, I would say that the leaves are green, but with a dash of purple added. The thirteenth-century name of 'thunder-clover' might refer to the leaf colour or to the belief that bugle brought thunderstorms. There is a naturally occurring sport with white flowers, whose leaves are bright green, and there is a very popular garden variety with deep-bronze leaves and rich purple flowers.

There was a saying, quoted in many herbals, that a person who had bugle and sanicle to hand would need neither physician nor surgeon. Bugle leaves, or the juice from them, would heal cuts and wounds and was 'wonderful in curing all manner of ulcers and sores', according to Culpeper. He went on to say: 'if the virtues of it make you fall in love with it (as they will if you be wise) keep a syrup of it to take inwardly, and an ointment and plaster of it to use outwardly, always by you'. I would happily use it 'outwardly', but would think twice about 'inwardly'.

∾ Self-heal

Looking similar to bugle, but flowering slightly later, is self-heal (*Prunella vulgaris*), common in short grass, on wasteland and in permanent pasture. It is a close relative of bugle and also a wound herb. A well-known medical herbalist told me that, when helping a friend to move house, he shut his thumb in a car door, injuring it quite badly. He noticed self-heal growing in his friend's lawn, so picked some, chewed it slightly to get the juices flowing, applied it to his thumb and wrapped a clean handkerchief around it. Each time he returned with another load of furniture, he replaced the makeshift poultice, and by the end of the day it was almost completely healed.

Bugle and self-heal are often confused, but bugle flowers are bluer and are carried in a taller spike. Self-heal's purple flowers are in a compact head with a pair of leaves immediately below it. Bugle's stem-leaves are sessile, while self-heal's are stalked. And for the really keen botanists: both have square stems; but bugle has hairs on only two sides, while self-heal is hairy all round.

Native to Europe, self-heal has spread to North America, and in the north-east the Algonquin, Mohegan and others give an infusion of it for fevers and sore throats. Gerard wrote:

> A decoction of Prunell made with wine and water, does join together and make whole and sound all wounds both inward and outward, even as Bugle does ... To be short, it serves for the same that Bugle does, and in the world there are not two better wound herbs, as has been often proved.

As with bugle, I often use self-heal leaves on cuts, but do not take it internally without direction from a qualified herbalist.

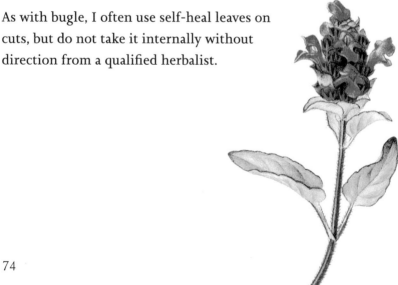

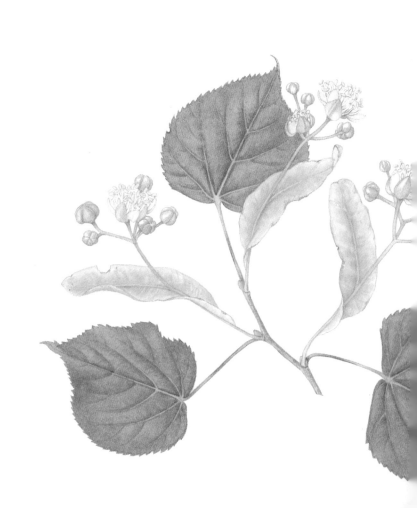

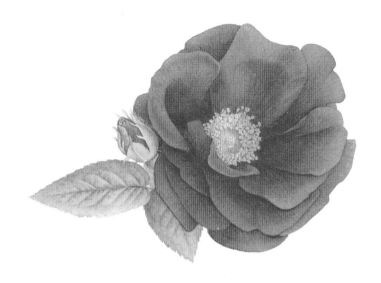

Early summer

Gather ye rosebuds while ye may

ROBERT HERRICK (1591–1674),
'To the Virgins, to Make Much of Time'

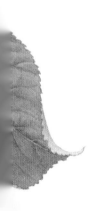

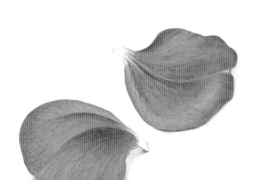

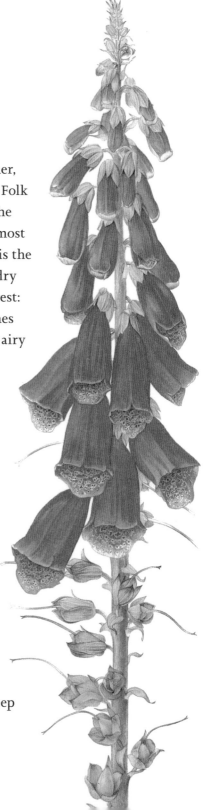

As spring blossoms into summer, herbalists become very busy. Folk tradition and writers down the ages all agree that herbs are at their most potent just before flowering, so now is the time to gather leaves and flowers to dry for use out of season. I love this harvest: in summer my house is full of bunches of herbs hanging up to dry in warm, airy places.

❧ Common foxglove

In early summer, the tall spires of foxglove flowers (*Digitalis purpurea*) begin to open. Foxglove grows in woodland clearings and more open habitats all over western Europe. The drooping, purple-magenta bells, arranged on one side of the stem, are perfectly made for bees to collect nectar in, while incidentally pollinating the flower. I never tire of watching bumblebees land on the projecting lower lip and crawl deep into the interior, making the bell buzz and vibrate while they work. The dark-purple spots inside, each surrounded by a white halo, may be there to guide insects in, or to warn of foxglove's poisonous nature. Legend, however, had it that the spots were the fingerprints of elves, who slipped the bells onto foxes' paws so that they could sneak up to hencoops undetected.

The connection with foxes and gloves goes back a long way. The Old English name was *foxes glofa* and many of foxglove's vernacular names suggest links with fairies or goblins. Foxglove had no scientific name until 1542, when the German botanist and physician Leonhart Fuchs coined *Digitalis*, a Latinised version of its German common name *Fingerhut*, meaning 'thimble'. As children, we used to slip the bells onto our fingers as make-believe thimbles. We did not know that all parts of the plant are poisonous. The ancient herbalists did not mention foxglove as a medicine – perhaps because it is uncommon in Greece and Italy – and this may account for the lack of a scientific name until so late.

Despite being so poisonous, foxglove found a place in English folk medicine, and was used externally to heal wounds and sores, and internally as an emetic and a purge. In 1756, John Hill wrote that it 'was more known among the country people than in the [apothecary's] shop' and that it often worked 'with a very hurtful violence' and was 'too rough for any but those who are very hardy'. But its main application was in the treatment of dropsy – tissues swollen with excess fluid, often a sign of heart failure. Treating such a serious condition was a gamble. If the physician administered the correct dose, foxglove worked quickly and well; if not, the patient died.

Having learned about this unpredictable folk medicine, in 1785 William Withering made a study of 158 cases of dropsy treated with an infusion of foxglove leaves, and realised how critical the dosage was. Rather than simply a diuretic, digitalis slows and strengthens the heart, which in turn stimulates the kidneys to expel excess fluid. But the wrong dose would stop the heart altogether. Today, Withering's work is regarded as the beginning of modern pharmacology, when 'active principles' were separated out and applied individually as treatments. Digitalis contains four glucosides, three of which have powerful effects on the heart. Of these, only one, digoxin, is used in conventional medicine today. *Digitalis lanata*, a close relative of common foxglove, was cultivated in northern Europe for the extraction of drugs. When, during the Second World War, supplies became unavailable, the County Herb Committees asked Women's Institutes all over Britain to collect common foxgloves as a replacement.

Foxglove is definitely not for home use as a medicine, but is a handsome addition to the garden, either as one of the many garden varieties or in its wild form. It obligingly produces huge quantities of seed – 1–2 million per plant, it is said – so foraging for some seeds from wild plants is excusable. The seeds require light to germinate, so I leave them uncovered. Plants will make a rosette of leaves the first year, then flower the second year and die, so it is worth sowing fresh seed annually, at least for the first two years.

∾ Chamomiles

The ancient Egyptians thought very highly of chamomile,
according to Galen. In fact, some authorities say they
dedicated it to the sun. Whether or not this is true,
chamomile has certainly been a trusted favourite for a very
long time. Its name is derived from Greek words meaning
'ground' and 'apple', as it grows close to the ground and
its leaves smell of apples. This fragrance is released when
the plant is trodden on, so chamomile became popular for
green paths in Elizabethan gardens. The saying was: 'Like
a chamomile bed – the more it is trodden, the more it will
spread.' Chamomile lawns and seats are nowadays planted
with the non-flowering variety 'Treneague'. Gardeners
believed that chamomile would revitalise other garden
plants, so called it 'the plants' physician'.

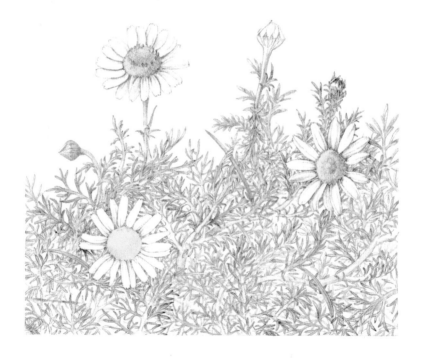

Common chamomile (*Chamaemelum nobile*) – which I always think of as the true chamomile – is native to western Europe. It has several related lookalikes, all with feathery leaves and daisy-like flowers. One, aptly called 'stinking chamomile', smells unpleasant and is strongly emetic. Another, scentless mayweed, speaks for itself. Of those growing wild in Britain, only three have *pleasantly* aromatic leaves. Corn chamomile, which has white fuzzy undersides to its leaves, is not prescribed medicinally. The other two – scented mayweed (*Matricaria chamomilla*, also called 'German' or 'wild' chamomile) and the common (or 'Roman') chamomile – are used more or less interchangeably, despite having slightly different constituent compounds. The ancient Egyptians were probably using wild chamomile, which is native as far east as India.

German chamomile has apple-green leaves with a stronger apple scent. Tests have shown that drinking infusions of German chamomile tea reduces the ability to absorb iron, but less so than consuming ordinary black tea. Common chamomile has grey-green leaves and long-stemmed single flowers. It tends to form mats. Its natural habitat is on light, sandy soils, especially in tightly grazed or frequently mown areas, such as village greens and commons, or in the clearings of the New Forest known as 'lawns'. A cricket-loving botanist friend tells me that it is sometimes found on cricket pitches, as the summer mowing and rolling replicates the grazing and trampling it needs to flourish. Chamomile is declining in Britain now, and is only found wild in a few areas of southern England; so please grow your own or buy the dried herb, rather than foraging from the wild.

Both common and German chamomile are relaxing and calming to the digestive and nervous systems, and are gentle enough for children's ailments, though you should always take medical advice before introducing herbs to children. In Beatrix Potter's tale, Peter Rabbit's mother put him to bed with a spoonful of chamomile tea after he had eaten too many stolen lettuces and only narrowly escaped from Mr McGregor. Chamomiles are anti-inflammatory, relaxant and sedative, as well as cleansing and cooling to the skin. Chamomile oil – which in German chamomile is a startling blue colour – makes for a de-stressing, calming massage: use two drops to five drops of carrier oil.

Seventeenth-century herbals suggested massaging with ointment made with chamomile and rose petals, or adding chamomile to the bathwater to 'take away weariness and ease pains'. And down the ages it has been a beauty treatment, too. An infusion made with a handful of chamomile flowers (or several chamomile teabags) in a jug of boiling water can be used – when cooled a little – as a final rinse for fair hair. A modern French herbal suggests boiling chamomile flowers in milk to make a hand lotion. And cooled chamomile teabags are a good compress for tired eyes and also for insect bites and stings.

Chamomile tea is made with dried flowers, using one teaspoonful to each cup. It is important to cover the infusion while it brews, or the volatile oils will be lost with the steam. If you find the taste too bitter, try adding a little honey, or some heather or lime flowers. Such an infusion, or tisane, will soothe anxiety and relax the body. However, chamomile tea is also diuretic – strong infusions were a treatment for kidney stones – so don't be surprised if, as a friend once complained, 'It puts you to sleep and then wakes you up to go to the bathroom!'

∿ Sage

When I first moved into my house some forty years ago, one of the first bushes I planted in the garden was common sage. I love its aromatic silvery leaves and the splendid spires of purple flowers in summer. The bees love it, too, which is always a bonus. I clip it over after flowering to keep it bushy, but can never bear to throw all the trimmings onto the compost heap, so I dry some for the kitchen and plant others as cuttings. Sage is short-lived but takes very easily from cuttings, so I have had a constant succession of sage bushes ever since. Sage belongs to the *Salvia* genus – about nine hundred species, many of which are prized as garden plants excellent for pollinators. The newly fashionable antioxidant 'superfood' chia seed comes from a Mexican species, *Salvia hispanica*.

Common sage (*Salvia officinalis*) is native to Mediterranean regions, but is the species most commonly grown for culinary and medicinal use worldwide. There is pollen evidence that the Egyptians were growing it in their physic gardens in 1224 BCE, and it appears in all the medieval lists of 'necessary herbs' to grow. It was – and still is – important as a culinary herb, especially good with pork or poultry. In our house, you couldn't possibly have roast chicken without sage and onion stuffing. In a 1393 guide to household management, the 'Goodman of Paris' writes of sage-water finger bowls; flavouring wine with a mixture of sage, ginger and bay leaves; and using a sage steam inhalation to cure toothache. Sage mouthwash has long been a remedy for mouth ulcers or sore gums, and many old texts such as *The Queen's Closet Opened* (1696) recommended cleaning the teeth with a sage leaf. In my childhood, Romany people were rumoured to use a mixture of sage and salt as a toothpowder.

Sage-leaf tea, sometimes with a little vinegar and honey added, was advised in old household books and herbals alike as a gargle for sore throats, laryngitis and tonsillitis. Sage contains thujone and antibacterial phenolic acids and is powerfully antiseptic, especially against *Staphylococcus aureus*, a frequent cause of sore throats. You could also drink an infusion to combat colds and fevers. Sage tea was thought to aid the digestion, too, and the leaves were made into a poultice for sprains. It is unsafe to drink sage-leaf tea regularly for more than a week or two at a time, as large amounts of thujone can be toxic. Medicinal doses of sage should not be taken during pregnancy.

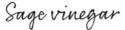

Sage vinegar

Roughly chop clean sage leaves, put into a jar and cover with cider vinegar or white wine vinegar. I use about 50g (2oz) fresh herb to 600ml (1 pint) vinegar.

Cover and allow to stand somewhere cool and dark for two weeks, shaking daily.

Strain through a sieve (strainer) lined with muslin (cheesecloth) and squeeze the cloth to get every drop of goodness out.

Pour the vinegar into a clean bottle, label and date.

I use a teaspoonful diluted in warm water as a gargle for sore throats, or soak a cloth in neat, hot vinegar as a compress for sprains.

In A Curious Herbal (1739), Elizabeth Blackwell wrote that 'the leaves and flowers are used as good for all diseases of the head and nerves. They are much used in all sorts of fevers, in tea or in posset drink.' Sage even calmed 'the shaking palsy' (probably Parkinson's disease). Nowadays its oestrogenic properties are thought to help with painful periods and hot flushes at the menopause. I found it best to chill the tea before drinking it for flushes.

In his 1607 The Englishman's Doctor, Sir John Harington listed sage's many medicinal benefits and commented (in rhyme) on its scientific and common names, Salvia (cognate with the Latin for 'save') and sage:

In Latin takes the name of safety,
In English is rather wise than crafty

The list of virtues claimed for sage is very long, reflected
by a Latin saying which translates as 'Why should a man
die whilst he has sage in his garden?' Or, as diarist John
Evelyn wrote, perhaps sarcastically, 'the assiduous use of
it is to render one immortal'. Certainly, in the eighteenth
century, it was said that the Chinese valued it so highly that
they traded three quantities of their finest tea for one of
European sage.

✍ Parsley

On the subject of parsley (*Petroselinum crispum*), Pliny wrote
in about 75 CE: 'Parsley is universally popular, for sprigs of it
are found swimming in draughts of milk everywhere in the
country, and in sauces it enjoys a popularity all its own.' He
went on to praise parsley's efficacy for a variety of ailments,
especially urinary, renal and uterine conditions. He said that
a poultice of parsley and bread would soothe spots and skin
eruptions – a view shared by some modern writers – and
that leaves pounded with water would relieve mouth ulcers.
Parsley is popular in folk medicine as a breath-freshener,
said even to eliminate 'garlic breath'. Sadly, tests appear to
indicate that the effect is temporary.

There are many medieval recipes for parsley dishes. In
1354, a huge seed order for the royal palace at Rotherhithe
included a staggering 14 lbs of parsley seed 'for sowing in the

King's garden in February'.
That much seed (equivalent
to 6.35kg) would plant about
an acre! Along with other herbs
like hyssop and sage, parsley was often
specified in accounts for royal gardens
and the 'cellarer's gardens' which served
the monasteries. Covent Garden, known
in 1200 as 'the garden of the Abbey and
Convent', was just one of several gardens
providing food and medicines for the
community of Westminster Abbey. We
should remember that these gardens fed
and treated not only the monastic community itself, but a
much larger population, including any associated satellite
houses and convents, the lay people working there, the sick
and destitute they cared for, and often many visitors, too. The
gardens also provided strewing herbs and hay for the latrines,
wash-houses and refectory. Royal and aristocratic households
had similar requirements.

Parsley is thought to be native in southern Europe, but
has naturalised around the world's temperate regions. It
has been cultivated in Britain since antiquity, occasionally
escaping into the wild. Many other similar-looking plants
have attracted 'parsley' names, such as 'bur-parsley' and 'cow
parsley', but only the true parsley has that characteristic
smell. 'Fool's parsley' is so called because, despite looking
superficially similar, it is poisonous. In fact, it has darker,
more finely divided leaves and an unpleasant smell when
crushed. It is safer to grow your own parsley, rather than

risk foraging a dangerous substitute. Many garden varieties of parsley have been developed, with flat or curled leaves. As a child, I only knew the frilly-leaved type and, seeing the flat-leaved sort for sale in French and Spanish markets, thought they were selling carrot tops. Parsley is hard to germinate – so much so that the seed was said to go to the Devil and back nine times before starting to grow. It was also supposed to thrive only where the woman of the house wore the trousers.

Parsley contains vitamins A and C, iron, potassium and calcium, so is nutritious, as well as tasty. Banckes's 1525 *Herbal* says 'it multiplies greatly a man's blood ... it comforts the heart and the stomach' – sentiments echoed by many later authors. There is also universal agreement among herbalists that parsley is diuretic and helps to expel uric acid, stones and gravel from the kidneys. During the First World War, parsley tea was given to the men in the trenches suffering with kidney problems resulting from dysentery. And parsley tea was often prescribed in English folk medicine for 'bladder troubles'.

Parsley's other main virtue is in women's medicine. It tones the uterine muscles, and helps to ease menstruation and to expel the afterbirth. For this reason, it is not recommended to take medicinal doses during pregnancy – in fact, there are records that at one time it was given to encourage abortion. As ever, you should consult your doctor, though nibbling a parsley garnish is probably fine, and may even contribute to blood iron levels.

I have always been slightly confused about marjoram and oregano. Writers ever since the ancient Greeks have added to the muddle by using different names for the same plant and the same name for different plants. The rather elastic spelling used in the past doesn't help either. What it boils down to is a related group of aromatic plants (Theophrastus classified them as under-shrubs) called the *Origanum* genus, from Greek words meaning 'mountain' and 'joy'. Within this genus are several species used in cooking and sometimes in medicine. Since classical times they have been important in perfumery, too, used to make chaplets and garlands and as strewing herbs. The two best-known members of the genus are sweet (or knotted) marjoram and wild marjoram, also called 'oregano' and 'pot marjoram', and even (by Gerard) 'organy'.

Sweet marjoram (*Origanum majorana*) originates in the Mediterranean area, but has been cultivated elsewhere for centuries. It has been found in the garlands of Egyptian mummies of the first century CE, and both Pliny and Dioscorides wrote that it was well known in ancient Egypt, too. The Romans said that the best and most fragrant plants came from Cyprus. Physicians of the time gave an infusion for irregular periods, strangury (difficulty in passing urine) and dropsy, and mixed the leaves with honey for bruises and with wax for sprains. From Roman times until quite recently, the dried, powdered leaves have been included in 'sneezing mixtures' (snuff) to clear the head.

There was an equally long history of making marjoram tea to relieve colds and to soothe the nerves.

Wild marjoram (*Origanum vulgare*), which is native in much of Europe, including Britain, is such a useful plant that it has been grown in gardens since at least 1350. It is taller and more robust than its sweet cousin, with purplish stems and larger leaves. It grows in rough grassland on calcareous soils and flowers later than sweet marjoram. A stand of wild marjoram in flower is a lovely late-summer sight, surrounded by butterflies and bees. In the sixteenth century, healers gave wild marjoram infusions for indigestion, 'gnawing of the stomach', respiratory conditions and many other ailments. It was so useful that early settlers took it with them to New England, where it has since naturalised.

Both wild and sweet marjoram were thought to be good treatments for bites, stings and poisoning, though far and away their best-loved attribute is their taste, which gives the characteristic

flavour to Mediterranean cookery. Many authors have called
the taste 'warming'. When on field trips in Mediterranean
countries, or in lime-rich areas
of Britain, I look out for one
or other marjoram to add
to my lunchtime salad or
sandwich. Both species, and
some other relatives, are used
interchangeably, rather as their
names sometimes are.

∾ Yarrow

Yarrow (*Achillea millefolium*)
was the first wildflower I really
engaged with as a child, noting
that some flowers were white, some
blushed pink, and others in shades of
pale lilac, too. I always loved its confetti
flowers and leaves like miniature ferns.
Years later I learned that great Achilles was
supposed to have used it to heal his soldiers'
wounds during the Trojan War, which
accounted for its scientific name. A tenth-
century Old English manuscript (actually a translation of the
fourth-century *Herbarium* of Pseudo-Apuleius, which itself
drew on Roman sources) repeated the story, and went on to
say: 'For wounds which are made with iron, take this same
wort, pounded with grease; lay it to the wounds; it purges

and heals the wounds.' More than five hundred years later, Banckes's *Herbal* repeated the entry almost word for word.

I love this chain of knowledge stretching back into history, but it isn't all scholarly borrowing. Alongside the written herbals is a long oral tradition of ordinary people applying yarrow to stop bleeding and heal cuts, indicated by such common names as 'carpenter's grass' and 'staunchweed'. It is hard to believe that people would give it those names or keep using it if it didn't help. Chinese traditional medicine also healed wounds with a poultice of fresh yarrow leaves. In Europe, yarrow was employed to stop bleeding both externally (with ointments and poultices) and internally (with infusions and decoctions). Another country name, 'nosebleed', is more confusing. In the sixteenth century, some authorities recommended gently inserting yarrow leaves into the nostrils to stop bleeding. Others suggested that the same action would *cause* a nosebleed, in order to relieve 'megrim' (migraine).

Yarrow tea was also well known as a fever treatment, especially for feverish colds or flu. A hot infusion of the flowering tops causes sweating, which lowers the temperature and helps eliminate toxins. A modern herbalist recommends a tea made of equal parts of dried elderflowers, peppermint and yarrow leaves as an excellent treatment in the early stages of flu. I put a teaspoonful of the mixture into a cup of boiling water and, if nothing else, it reminds me of summer. The alkaloids that yarrow contains, and its action in bringing blood to the skin surface, help to lower blood pressure. In the 1920s and 1930s in Russia, a decoction of elderflowers and yarrow was drunk to relieve skin conditions like eczema.

Yarrow also had a long-standing reputation as an anti-inflammatory, which modern research appears to confirm, due to the salicylates it contains. The tenth-century *Lacnunga* prescribes 'a good bathing' for inflammation: a pleasant-sounding warm bath infused with ivy, yarrow, honeysuckle leaves and cowslips.

As well as its medicinal value, yarrow was thought to have magical properties. It protected you from evil, or divined your future. The Chinese I Ching (Yijing) used yarrow stalks for divination, and an old East Anglian rhyme neatly combines medicine with magic:

> Yarroway, yarroway, bear a white blow [flower]
> If my love loves me, my nose will bleed now.

Yarrow is common everywhere in the wild, so was not generally grown in gardens, except in physic gardens. It is stoloniferous and seeds freely, so can become a nuisance; but there are now many garden varieties with richly coloured flowers that are very popular both with gardeners and bees.

∾ Lime

In prehistoric Britain, small-leaved lime (Tilia cordata) was the dominant tree species in the southern Wildwood. It is still found in the south, but in much smaller numbers. Britain's other native species, large-leaved lime (Tilia platyphyllos) is, and always was, much less common. However, the hybrid between the two native trees is everywhere, frequently

planted as a street tree. It is called, aptly
enough, 'common lime' (*Tilia x europaea*).
All three have wonderfully fragrant
flowers beloved of bees – in fact, you often
hear or smell a flowering lime tree before you
see it.

With the heady scent of its blossom and its
heart-shaped leaves, lime was 'the tree of love', and lime
walks and what one writer called 'brave summer houses
and banqueting arbors' were popular garden features from
medieval times. Brave is perhaps the right word, as limes
attract honeydew-producing aphids, so sweethearts dallying
under a lime tree risked becoming rather sticky, as anyone
who has unwisely parked their car under a lime tree will
know. Some people thought the honeydew a bonus, making
lime leaves taste like sweetened lettuce. I won't be adding
them to my salads, but might try an idea proposed by
a nineteenth-century French chemist. He claimed that
lime fruits, pounded with dried lime flowers, tasted like
chocolate.

Lime trees have attracted a variety of vernacular names,
some of which are embedded in place names such as Linwood,
Lindrick or Lyndhurst, all from *lin* or *linde*, the Old English for
'lime tree'. Lime was often coppiced for thin poles, and some
coppice stools are enormous, possibly dating back several
thousand years. The timber is not very strong, but is excellent
for carving, so long as it is properly seasoned. Theophrastus
noted how easy it was to work, and the famous English
master carver Grinling Gibbons (1648–1721) favoured it for his
stunningly intricate carvings for churches and grand houses.

Our forebears also made use of the fibrous inner bark, or 'bast'. It is white, moist and tough, excellent for twisting into ropes and halters. Lime bast is diuretic, so was sometimes given to treat kidney disorders, too.

But it is the flowers that were most important medicinally. Culpeper wrote that a distillation of lime flowers and 'lily convally' was good for 'griping in the guts'. I suppose he means lily of the valley (*Convallaria majalis*), whose red berries are poisonous – I would be nervous that the flowers might be, too. However, an infusion of lime flowers alone, famous in France as *tilleul*, has long been a trusted treatment for nervous tension, headache and insomnia. The blossoms contain bioflavonoids, which have a reputation for lowering blood pressure. I often make a tea with dried lime flowers, dried rose petals and fresh lemon balm leaves as a relaxing bedtime drink.

✤ Roses

In April 2008, I was botanising at the foot of the Boraldai mountain range in Kazakhstan. That early in the year there were wonderful wild tulips and other flowering bulbs, but not much else in bloom. Then, on a dark scree slope, I spotted a wild rose in flower. It had primrose-yellow petals, deep-red filaments and a heavenly scent. Instantly transfixed, I spent a long time with my chilly hands cupped round the flowers, inhaling the perfume. Such is the eternal allure of roses. I have no doubt that our prehistoric ancestors buried their noses in roses, too.

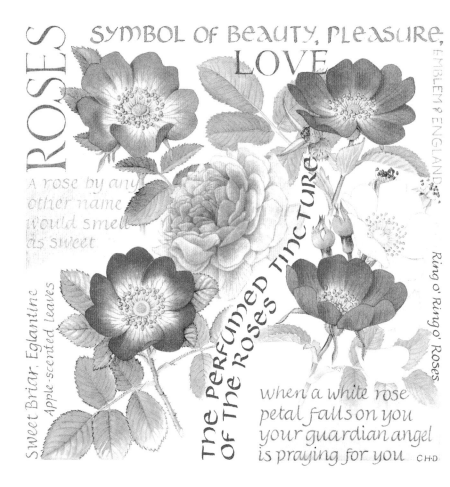

ROSES

SYMBOL OF BEAUTY, PLEASURE, LOVE

EMBLEM ♀ ENGLAND

A rose by any other name would smell as sweet

Sweet Briar, Eglantine. Apple-scented leaves

THE PERFUMED TINCTURE OF THE ROSES

Ring o' Ringo' Roses

when a white rose petal falls on you your guardian angel is praying for you CHD

Roses appear in wall paintings at Knossos Palace, Crete, dating from 2000 BCE, and were well known to the ancient Egyptians and in ancient India, too. They were brought into cultivation early on – especially in Persia and China – and it is now quite challenging to trace their origins, after centuries of hybridisation. In ancient Greece, Theophrastus wrote about their cultivation and uses. His book *Concerning Odours* describes how perfumes were made, and their effects on the body. He said that rose was 'specially helpful against strangury', and was 'good against lassitude'. He described how perfumes were applied externally in poultices or plasters to heal internal ills. Aromatherapy has deep roots!

In the twelfth century, Abbess Hildegard of Bingen wrote that any medication would be more effective with the addition of even a little rose, because of its 'good virtues'. She also advised putting fresh rose petals on the eyelids on waking, to clear the sight. Rose water appears in many medieval treatments for heart conditions and in eye salves. In 1607, one 'A.T.', a 'practitioner in physic', recommended a silk pad filled with rose petals, saffron, oil of mace and civet. He said you should 'apply it to the region of the heart, and it will do you marvellous much good'. In the seventeenth century, rose juice was prescribed for the ears, sores in the mouth, the gums, the stomach, uterus and rectum, as a gargle for the tonsils, to induce sleep, cure headaches and dispel nausea – an impressive list.

Roses were made into a variety of preparations. The petals do impart their perfume easily, and the 'rose oil' of ancient writers was often a sun-infused oil, made as described by Pliny (see recipe below). This was, he wrote, a process known at the time of the Trojan War and mentioned by Homer. Distilling the essential oil – 'attar of roses' – is a more complicated business. It takes thirty roses to produce a single drop of oil, which is why it is so costly. Today it is added to perfume and toiletries, while herbalists and aromatherapists apply it to encourage self-care and in cases of grief.

Rose petals keep their perfume well when dried, so were used to sweeten linen cupboards and to freshen rooms. Distilled rose water gave a delectable taste to junketing dishes, cakes, sauces and many other pleasant treats.

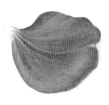

Pliny's rose oil

rose petals 'steeped with oil or wine in a glass vessel in the sunshine'

Loosely fill a glass jar with clean, dry rose petals – the more fragrant the better. If you use red petals, the oil may turn a lovely pink. Pliny recommended cutting off the white 'nails', as they can cause mould. (I have tried it both ways and he was right, of course.) Top up the jar with light olive or sunflower oil, making sure the petals are all submerged, and stand it in the sun for two to four weeks.

Once the petals have lost their colour, remove them and add fresh petals.

Leave in the sun for another two to four weeks. (For a more strongly scented oil, repeat once or twice more.)

Strain carefully, discarding any watery liquid at the bottom, as this can spoil the oil. Pour into clean bottles and label.

This recipe also works with dried rose petals, which avoids any risk of spoilt oil. And if you live somewhere without reliable sunshine, it can be made by standing the jar in gently simmering water for two hours, and repeating with new petals.

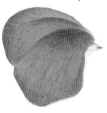

And true Turkish Delight is probably still the most famous rose-scented confection today.

The roses most often grown for their medicinal properties were *Rosa* x *damascena* and *Rosa gallica officinalis*, known as the 'apothecary's rose'. Every monastery garden would cultivate those, and by the later Middle Ages they were grown commercially for the production of oil and rose water. Native wild roses were not much valued in medicine, apart from their fruits, or hips.

✺ Balm

Balm (*Melissa officinalis*), also called 'lemon balm' because of its lemon-scented leaves, is a cottage-garden favourite originating in southern Europe, but now grown in gardens everywhere. It is sometimes found growing wild near habitation, having seeded from gardens. Classical physicians knew it well and thought it good for a long list of conditions, including skin sores, indigestion, dysentery, inflammation and even dog bites: Dioscorides says the leaves are good for 'the scorpion-smitten and the dog-bitten'. Another name for this lovely plant is 'bee-balm', as bees love it – another good reason for growing it. Its scientific name *Melissa* comes from the Greek for honey-bee. Pliny writes: 'no flower gives them greater pleasure', and says that rubbing balm over their hives will stop the bees from flying away. He also claims that the leaves are a good treatment for bee stings, which is handy.

The deliciously lemon-flavoured leaves, picked just before flowering, make a lovely addition to wine cups and to fish dishes. Medieval recipes for uplifting cordials often included balm, and it is still an ingredient of both Bénédictine and Chartreuse liqueurs. For generations, balm was highly valued for its effect on the mind. Tenth-century Persian physician Avicenna said balm 'makes the heart merry'; and in the seventeenth century, John Evelyn wrote 'balm is sovereign for the brain, strengthening the memory, and powerfully chasing away melancholy'. The fresh herb and essential oil are still used today for nervous headaches, depression and insomnia.

Scientific investigations show that an infusion of leaves significantly benefits mood and cognition, and has relaxing properties and an anti-spasmodic action on the digestive system. Applied topically to cold sores, balm has an anti-viral effect, reducing recovery time. The Romans prescribed balm to promote menstruation, so don't take it if you are pregnant. The leaves lose their volatile oils in drying, so are best used fresh to make an uplifting tea. I sometimes pot up a small clump of balm to bring indoors for fresh leaves out of season.

∾ Mints

A ninth-century writer said that there were as many varieties of mint as there were sparks from Vulcan's furnace. There certainly is a bewildering number of hybrids and varieties on offer today, with coloured, variegated or differently scented leaves. All derive from the *Mentha* genus of aromatic, moisture-loving wild plants that have been familiar in Eurasia and Africa throughout history. It is such a delightful surprise when unexpectedly treading on some water mint by the riverside, and our prehistoric ancestors can't have failed to notice it either. The smell of mint refreshes our spirits, and its flavour gives a zest to our food. Mints were valued in ancient Egypt, as well as in traditional Chinese and Ayurvedic medicine. Classical physicians gave very long lists of mints' medicinal virtues and prescribed them to treat everything from chilblains to snake bite and cholera. Folk medicine everywhere gave infusions of various mint species to treat colds and fevers, as well as for the digestion and for inflammatory skin conditions.

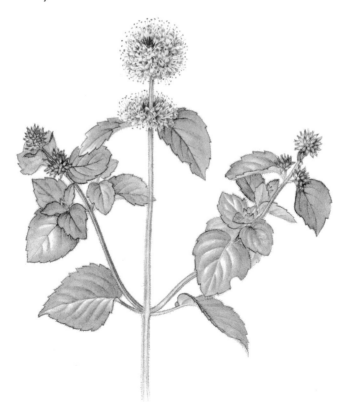

The mints most often grown in gardens are spearmint (*Mentha spicata*), pennyroyal (*Mentha pulegium*) and peppermint (*Mentha x piperita*), which is a cross between water mint and spearmint. This hybrid was first recorded towards the end of the seventeenth century, but must have occurred in the wild frequently before that. We know peppermint best today as a digestive aid, drinking it as a tea after meals or sucking it as a peppermint-flavoured sweet. It does settle a queasy stomach, though I find it diuretic, too. Scientific research confirms that peppermint oil has an anti-spasmodic effect on what Abbess Hildegard of Bingen called 'hot intestines'. It is particularly beneficial in irritable bowel syndrome. Peppermint's volatile oil is mainly menthol, which is antibacterial, anaesthetic and anti-inflammatory. Applied externally it is proven to help with muscle pain, and it is included in inhalants to treat colds and catarrh, along with aromatics like camphor and eucalyptus. Effective though it is, peppermint oil should be used with caution, in small doses, and always diluted. Do not use it externally on young children, as there have been isolated cases where it has caused breathing difficulties.

Of course, toothpastes and mouthwashes are flavoured with peppermint, not to mention many favourite sweets, chocolates and desserts. Personally I prefer the taste of spearmint to peppermint. It makes a lovely tea, which is very popular in the Middle East and North Africa. I first tried it on a rickety train to Marrakesh in 1974, dispensed by an elderly itinerant tea-seller with a huge brass kettle and a basket of mint on his back. In Britain, spearmint is the species we put in with our new potatoes and the first of the garden peas. And it is the one we use to make mint sauce. As soon as I was old enough to be trusted with scissors, I was sent out to collect mint from the garden for sauce to go with the Sunday roast lamb. We chopped the mint finely and mixed it with vinegar and sugar in a little white jug.

Pennyroyal is a creeping, often mat-forming, British native mint which smells of peppermint. Its specific name *pulegium* derives from *pulex*, Latin for 'flea', and it was always a popular insecticidal strewing herb. In 1818, Joseph Taylor noted that hot infusions of it were taken for 'inveterate coughs' and asthma. Although people have tended to use different mint species interchangeably, they do have different constituents. Unlike other mints, pennyroyal contains some volatile oils which can be toxic in excess, and it should be avoided, especially in pregnancy.

Mints have always been popular in gardens, though they are very invasive. The roots can creep a very long way. I have tried planting them in a bottomless bucket sunk into the soil, but they easily escaped. Perhaps an old chimney-pot would have been better, or a wide-gauge drainage pipe. Mints were always grown in monastic cellarer's gardens for food, medicines and for strewing – I wonder how they dealt with the invasive roots.

ᘒ Poppies

Some of the most flamboyant summer flowers are the poppies, though they are definitely not for medicinal use at home. Oriental poppies, with their huge flowers in a range of vibrant colours, can hardly be ignored in the garden, with what Ted Hughes called their 'carnival paper skirts'. But Britain's native, wild poppies, too, are stunning. The yellow horned poppy (*Glaucium flavum*) grows by the sea and has glaucous leaves, big yellow flowers and splendid long, curved seed pods – the 'horns' that give it its name. In 1677, John Aubrey wrote of it as 'squatmore' – 'squat' was an old name for a bruise – and reported that it was 'of wonderful effect for bruises'.

Europe's familiar scarlet common poppy (*Papaver rhoeas*) or 'corn rose' used to be common in cornfields, and still thrives in disturbed ground everywhere. It flourished in abundance when the battlefield of Waterloo was ploughed, and in Flanders after the First World War. The idea grew that it symbolised the blood of slaughtered soldiers. There was also the story of Ceres, the Roman goddess of agriculture. She neglected the crops and exhausted herself searching for her kidnapped daughter, until the gods took pity on her and gave her poppies to enable her to sleep and forget her distress. These stories combined to suggest the poppy as a symbol of remembrance.

However, the poppy most prescribed to relieve pain and promote sleep was the opium poppy (*Papaver somniferum*). It has been found in a Neolithic village excavation in Switzerland and in an ancient Egyptian tomb. The ancient

Greeks ate poppy buds as a purge. Pliny described in detail
the process of harvesting and processing the sap. He says
'it is not only a soporific, but if too large a dose is given
the sleep even ends in death. It is called opium.' The milky
sap contains alkaloids, including morphine and codeine –
both invaluable medicines when used properly, but deadly
when abused. Monks grew opium poppies in their physic
gardens and kept the opium locked up with other dangerous
narcotics, such as henbane, hemlock and mandrake. Opium
was given for eye conditions, as well as for pain relief,
according to Prospero Alpini, writing in the late 1500s.
A tincture of opium, known as 'laudanum', was a popular
analgesic for centuries, though it, too, was dangerously
addictive. Poppy seeds contain no opiates – though they
are occasionally contaminated with tiny amounts during
processing – and are still popular in baking today.

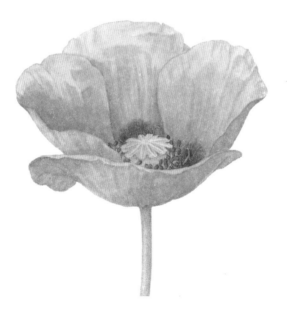

❧ Borage

Medieval gardeners considered borage (*Borago
officinalis*) another essential plant to grow,
harvesting its leaves for 'pottage' and 'salad'. All but
the youngest leaves are rather too bristly to eat raw, but can
be cooked like spinach or made into fritters. They taste like
cucumber and are rich in calcium and potassium. Modern
gardeners in temperate regions worldwide complain about
their borage seeding itself everywhere, but those glorious
blue flowers are as welcome to me as they are to the bees. It
does spread into the wild on roadsides and waste ground,
but never very far from human habitation. Its starry blue
petals with the white centre and column of dark anthers
are so attractive that cooks have been adding them to salads
and cold drinks for generations. And they are, of course, an
essential addition to summer cocktails such as a Pimm's.
As a young wife keen to impress her husband's business
associates, I used to freeze borage flowers in ice cubes for
their cocktails.

The ancient writers all knew borage, a native of southern
Europe, and all of them praised its leaves and flowers as a
treatment for melancholy. There was a Latin saying which
translates as 'I, borage, always bring courage'; and one of its
Welsh names means 'herb of gladness'. In the third (1628)
edition of his scholarly work on depression, *The Anatomy of
Melancholy*, Robert Burton included an allegorical frontispiece
illustrating aspects of the condition. Borage and hellebore
both appear, as 'the best medicine that e'er God made for this
malady, if well assayed'. Borage leaves have also been used, at

least since the time of Galen, to relieve colds and coughs in a hot infusion.

Recent research shows that borage seeds contain significant levels of essential fatty acids, including gamma-linolenic acid (GLA), believed by some to alleviate a whole range of conditions. Like its close relative comfrey, borage is thought to affect the sex hormones, increasing the production of milk in nursing mothers. This may account for its reputation as a remedy for menopausal and pre-menstrual symptoms. In the 1980s, borage was grown commercially for its GLA, until waste blackcurrant pulp was discovered to yield more GLA at lower cost.

❧ Evening primrose

Originating in North America, the beautiful evening primroses (Oenothera spp) light up summer evenings with their large, primrose-yellow flowers. Poet John Clare says it 'wastes its fair bloom upon the night', as the flowers open at dusk. In fact the blooms – 'almost as pale as moonbeams are' – attract night-flying insects to pollinate them. Evening primroses were first brought from Virginia to Padua in 1614 as a garden curiosity, and they have since naturalised in much of Europe and elsewhere. There were patches of them growing on dunes in Lancashire, said to be from seeds in ballast dumped by ships bringing cotton to Liverpool from the southern states of America. It certainly does seed freely, and likes poor soil.

The Navajo, Blackfoot and many other Native American peoples used various Oenothera species, making poultices of

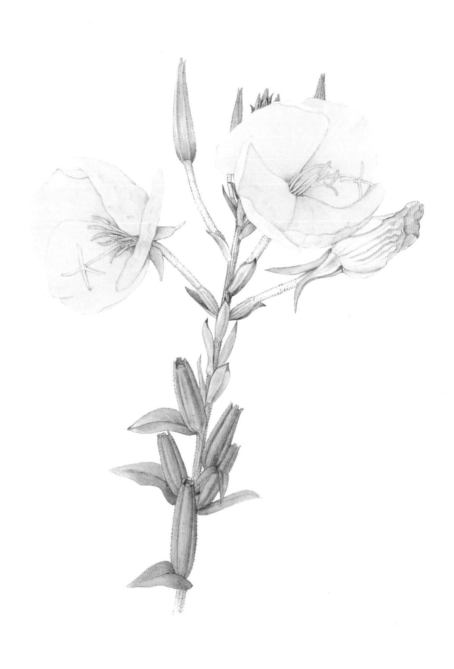

leaves or roots for painful rheumatic swellings, or treating venereal sores with dried, powdered leaves. It had ceremonial applications, too, and was mixed with tobacco and smoked to bring luck in hunting. Only one tribe, the Potawatomi, reported collecting the seeds, which they considered a valuable medicine; frustratingly, however, they did not record what for.

In fact, oil from the seeds is rich in GLA, and some have hailed evening primrose oil as a panacea, lowering cholesterol and blood pressure, and curing everything from multiple sclerosis and gastric problems to whooping cough and especially 'women's troubles'. The many scientific trials have unfortunately come up with conflicting results. The effect on eczema and dermatitis, pre-menstrual tension, menopausal hot flushes and breast pain is still debated. The oil was found to relieve the pain of rheumatoid arthritis, but only in large doses. Combined with other essential fatty acids, it has helped significantly in attention deficit hyperactivity disorder (ADHD). Because of its possible anti-coagulant properties, people on blood-thinning medication should avoid evening primrose oil. It should not be taken long term or during pregnancy, but if you suffer from PMT or menopausal symptoms, it might be worth checking with your doctor to see if commercially produced capsules, with the potentially dangerous substances extracted, could work for you.

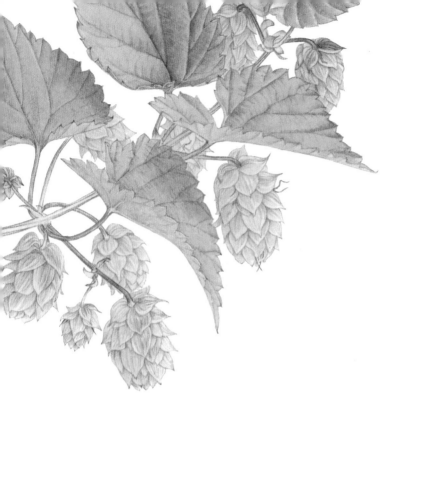
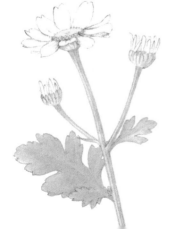

High summer

Now the fields are laughing

ANON.,
manuscript of Benediktbeuern
(thirteenth century)

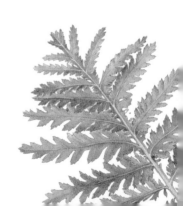

❧ Nasturtiums

Many of us as children were given nasturtium seeds to sow: they grow quickly and produce large plants with showy flowers – a perfect combination for novice gardeners. Nasturtiums spread into the wild in some places, but are killed off by the first frost. Early explorers brought back seeds from South America, and by 1597 John Gerard was writing excitedly that he had 'this rare and fair plant' in his own garden, grown from seed sent by a friend in Paris. It was such a recent introduction that he had 'no certain knowledge of [its] nature and virtues'. He would certainly have tried nibbling a leaf and have noticed its hot, peppery taste. In my childhood, we occasionally included shredded nasturtium leaves in salads and sandwiches, but more often we pickled the fruits as a substitute for capers. Adding those big orange or yellow flowers to salads is a relatively recent fashion, impossibly exotic for us in the buttoned-up 1950s.

Garden nasturtium is thought to act as a natural antibiotic that does not destroy the gut flora, as so many antibiotics do. Healers gave infusions of the leaves for bronchitis and

for urinary infections, and some modern herbalists still
do. Linnaeus gave it the scientific name of *Tropaeolum*, from
the Greek *tropaion*, the trophy tree on which the armour of
defeated enemies was displayed after a battle. Nasturtium
plants were commonly grown up supports, and the leaves
and flowers reminded Linnaeus of round shields and golden,
blood-streaked helmets. The woodcut illustrating nasturtium
in Gerard's *Herbal* shows it grown up a cane. I usually let
it scramble over a bank, or tumble from a wall-basket, but
perhaps I will try growing it up a support next summer
instead.

∾ Watercress

Nasturtium is in fact the scientific name for our European
native watercress and its close relatives. The name comes
from the Latin for 'twisted nose', on account of its pungency.
People have always valued watercress (*Nasturtium officinale*)
for its flavour, and Hippocrates recommended it as an
expectorant and stimulant. John Evelyn wrote disparagingly
of it in his 1699 essay on salads, saying it would 'nourish
little', though actually it is full of vitamins and minerals,
especially helpful for people convalescing after illness. Other
writers considered it powerful against scurvy and good for
the blood. It was always given to us as children if we looked a
little anaemic or lacklustre.

Watercress grows on the banks of fast-flowing streams,
especially chalk streams, and country people have
gathered it for generations − it is even mentioned in

Anglo-Saxon documents. By the eighteenth century, its nutritive value was recognised and large-scale collection began, and then cultivation. In the railway age, special 'watercress lines' brought the crop to London for sale by street vendors.

Gathering watercress in the wild can be dangerous. Medieval coroners' rolls record the deaths of many peasant women, drowned while collecting watercress and other herbs from river banks. And wild watercress is host to the liver fluke, which can cause serious liver damage if ingested. Better to enjoy the safe, cultivated watercress sold in shops. If you put a sprig or two into water they will readily take root and grow more shoots for you to enjoy.

☙ St John's wort

By midsummer, various kinds of
St John's wort (Hypericum spp) are
beginning to bloom. They all
have cheerful yellow flowers with
a characteristic 'powder puff'
of stamens in the centre.
Wort is the Old English
word for 'plant', but where
does St John come into it?
The theory is that, as the plant
was one of the magical herbs used
in pagan summer solstice rituals,
it was Christianised by linking it to

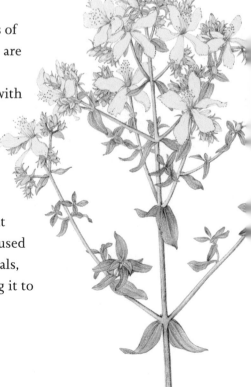

St John, whose feast day was three days later, on 24 June. That sounds perfectly reasonable, but doesn't take account of the Gregorian calendar reform. The old Julian calendar year was fractionally longer than the astrological year, and so, over the centuries, natural phenomena such as solstices and equinoxes crept out of alignment with calendar dates. In particular, this made calculating the date of Easter difficult, so reform was needed. Eventually, in 1582, Pope Gregory XIII decreed a change to a new calendar. To rectify the previous 'creep', ten days were dropped: 4 October was directly followed by 15 October. (Protestant Britain did not follow suit until 1752, when eleven days were dropped.) So, before the change, St John's Day fell even further away from the summer solstice. And yet there are records of the name 'St John's wort' as far back as the thirteenth century.

However, it is certain that the Hypericum genus has always been considered magical and medicinal. Some say that the scientific name comes from Greek words meaning 'above' and 'icon', suggesting that these protective flowers decorated sacred images in ancient festivals. It is a large genus, with species found all over the world. In Britain there are several native herbaceous species, as well as the shrubby tutsan, whose large, flat leaves smell pleasantly musky when dried. They were used as bookmarks, so the plant used to be called 'Bible-leaf'. I still use tutsan bookmarks. The species used in herbal medicine is perforate St John's wort (Hypericum perforatum), common in grassy places. Hold a leaf up to the light and you will see why 'perforate' is so apt: there are lots of transparent dots, which folklore claims are where the Devil pricked it in revenge for its powers of protection against evil. In fact, the dots are oil glands.

Roman physicians knew two kinds of 'hypericon' and recommended decoctions of their seeds for diarrhoea, bladder troubles, sciatica, fevers and spasms. Applied externally, the whole plant would treat burns, too. Gerard gave a detailed description of making a sun-infused oil for burns and wounds. In the 1960s, a fair-skinned student friend, staying with a family in the south of France, suffered a badly sunburned back. His hostess produced a bottle of alarmingly red oil, which cooled his skin and healed it without blistering. She told him that it was made from St John's wort steeped in olive oil in the sun – exactly as Gerard had described (see below). Scientific research confirms the efficacy of St John's wort oil both for wounds and for burns.

Today the best-known application of St John's wort is in treating depression, and there are many preparations containing hypericins extracted from the herb available over the counter. A great deal of research has been carried out into these herbal preparations, and the studies report excellent results in treating some forms of depression, with fewer side effects than conventional medication. However, they also found that St John's wort interacts with many other medications, and even interferes with oral contraceptives. So please consult a pharmacist or other health professional before taking St John's wort internally. St John's wort shouldn't be taken if you are pregnant, trying to get pregnant, or nursing.

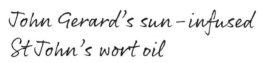

John Gerard's sun-infused St John's wort oil

'a most precious remedy'

Loosely fill a glass jar with lightly crushed leaves, flowers and seeds of St John's wort. Fill up the jar with olive oil, put on the lid and set in the hot sun for about two to three weeks.

Strain through a sieve (strainer) lined with muslin (cheesecloth).

Fill the jar with a fresh quantity of crushed herb (leaves, flowers and seeds) and pour the strained oil back in.

'Sun' it for another two or three weeks.

Strain again, discarding any watery juice at the bottom – this would cause the oil to deteriorate quickly. Pour into clean bottles and label.

It may have become 'an oil the colour of blood'; but don't worry if it is paler – it will still be useful for treating wounds, bruises and burns.

✇ Dropwort and meadowsweet

DROPWORT

A plant credited with curing gravel or kidney stones was
dropwort (*Filipendula vulgaris*). Culpeper explained that it was
so named 'because it gives ease to those that piss by drops'.
A European native plant, it grows on chalk or limestone
grassland; it has pinnate leaves – not unlike tansy leaves,
but tougher in texture. In England, the young leaves were
added to salads, but in Sweden were considered only fit for
pigs' fodder. Dropwort carries a head of small, creamy white,
six-petalled flowers in high summer, and the tiny buds are
a pretty pink. No wonder medieval gardeners grew it for its
beauty, as well as its healing virtues.

MEADOWSWEET

Dropwort's much better-known and more common relative,
meadowsweet (*Filipendula ulmaria*), flourishes in damp
meadows and riversides all over northern Europe and in
the east of North America. On a sultry summer's day you
often smell it before you see it, as the frothy, five-petalled
flowers have a powerful perfume. In Wales and in England,
a superstition persisted right up until the twentieth
century that if you fell asleep breathing their scent, you
might never wake up again. Archaeologists have found
evidence of quantities of meadowsweet in several Bronze
Age burials in Britain. The leaves have a slightly different
scent, and that difference is noted in another vernacular

name, 'courtship-and-matrimony', contrasting the sweetness of the flowers with the sharper, more antiseptic scent of the crushed leaves.

It was an ideal strewing herb, of course, said to be Elizabeth I's favourite. A writer of the time remarked that it lifted the spirits and delighted the senses, but did not cause headaches or put you off your food, as some strong scents could do. The smell reminds me of marzipan, but en masse can be a bit overwhelming. If you have a hand lens or magnifying glass, it's worth looking at the fruits of meadowsweet, the naked carpels 'crookedly turning or winding one with another, made into a fine little head', as Gerard wrote. I agree, they are delightful to see.

In the seventeenth century, it was said that a meadowsweet leaf 'gave a fine relish' to a glass of claret, while the flowers have been used for centuries to flavour drinks, especially mead. The plant was originally called 'mede-wort' or 'mede-sweet', possibly from this custom; but by 1530 the name was evolving into 'meadowsweet', reflecting its habitat, too.

An infusion of flowers promoted sweating, helpful in agues (fevers), especially malaria – which in the Middle Ages was endemic in Europe, including

Britain. In more recent times, folk healers gave women meadowsweet tea to treat anaemia. An infusion of the leaves is said to relieve headaches, and I gather some stems when the plant is in flower, to dry the leaves for winter use. Meadowsweet has been valued in medicine for a very long time. The Anglo-Saxons are known to have prescribed it, and there are records of people still collecting it in the early part of the twentieth century. A Board of Agriculture leaflet published during the First World War listed it as wanted by herbalists and pharmacists.

Meadowsweet is one source of salicylates, which are oxidised into salicylic acid in the digestive tract. First isolated by an Italian scientist in 1838, salicylic acid can be converted into acetylsalicylic acid – aspirin – and by 1899 the pharmaceutical company Bayer had begun production of this new and incredibly useful drug. The name 'aspirin' comes from *Spiraea*, the old botanical name for meadowsweet. However, herbalists point to the dangers of isolating active principles from herbs: aspirin can cause gastric bleeding, while meadowsweet itself also contains mucilage and tannins which protect against such damage. In fact, one of meadowsweet's 'virtues' is as a remedy for acid stomach.

∾ Willow

Salicylates were also isolated from the bark of white willow (*Salix alba*), so called because its pubescent leaves shimmer like silver when the wind blows. Mankind has known and

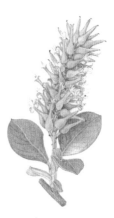

used willows since the beginning of history. There is a painting of a pollarded willow in an Egyptian tomb of about 1200 BCE, and many ancient scholars wrote about them. Because the bark is so bitter, willow became a symbol for those grieving for lost love, or 'wearing the green willow'. Poor Ophelia drowned while, fittingly, trying to hang garlands of wildflowers on a willow 'aslant a brook'.

Although using their twigs and timber for a great variety of different purposes, people did not generally distinguish between willow species as remedies. Healers prescribed the leaves and bark of several different species for pain relief, to treat cuts, stop diarrhoea and to cure fevers. In 1763, Rev. Edward Stone noticed that rheumatism and fever – and also willow trees – flourished in marshy areas. Believing that for all ailments 'their remedies lie not far from their causes', he began to experiment, giving a decoction of willow bark to fifty or so sufferers. His results were very encouraging, and have since been confirmed in modern clinical trials. Research also indicates that the whole herb does not damage the stomach to the same extent as aspirin alone. Although the research also shows that people with diabetes, or with liver or gastro-intestinal conditions, or who are taking anti-coagulant or blood-thinning medication should use willow with caution.

∾ Feverfew

Another plant which gardeners find invasive is feverfew (*Tanacetum parthenium*). All the books, even the medieval ones, say that it grows as a weed by walls, in odd corners and on waste ground. If it doesn't like your soil, you can treat it as an annual and grow new plants in pots each year for the pretty light-green foliage and bright-as-buttons flowers. It is one of several plants known by the country name of 'bachelor's buttons'. There are many garden varieties, with golden leaves or double flowers, but I like the simple, natural kind best.

Feverfew (or 'featherfew' as it was often called) originates in the Balkans and Turkey, but has been grown as a medicinal plant for centuries and often escapes into the wild. The ancients knew it – Dioscorides recommended it as an anti-inflammatory – and it appears in several Anglo-Saxon treatments for ulcers and skin sores. As its name suggests, it was given for feverish colds, among other things; but its main value was as an analgesic for headaches and rheumatic pain. Although the old physicians knew about migraine (or 'megrim', as they rather aptly called it), they did not prescribe feverfew as a treatment.

In the 1970s, following a newspaper report about a woman curing herself of chronic migraines by eating feverfew leaves, many sufferers rushed to try the remedy for themselves. Tests run by a specialist migraine clinic showed that a majority of patients experienced a significant reduction in the number and severity of attacks. Taken over several months, feverfew seemed to prevent the spasms in the tiny blood vessels supplying the brain which are thought to trigger migraines. Because of its action on the blood vessels, it is not recommended for people on blood-thinning medication.

Many people find that feverfew reduces their migraines, whether in tablet form or as fresh leaves, best eaten in sandwiches to mask its bitter taste. Unfortunately, further scientific research has proved inconclusive, and points to the possibility of side effects, such as mouth ulcers. On the other hand, many test patients reported *positive* side effects, including relief from depression. This confirms another historical use: several authors from Tudor times onwards say that feverfew is good for those 'who are troubled with melancholy or lowness of spirits'.

✆ Tansy

In medieval Europe, people ate 'tansies' – puddings or cakes made with the young leaves of tansy (*Tanacetum vulgare*) – at Easter time. Tansies were supposed to purge the bad humours engendered by a diet of salted fish during Lent. They are 'pleasant in taste', said one writer, 'and good for the stomach'. I tried it once and found it distinctly unpleasant. Tansy is native throughout most of Europe, including Britain, growing on waste ground and rough grassland; but it was brought into medieval gardens as much for its medicinal properties as for the

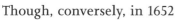

pot. Physicians prescribed
infusions of leaves or
seeds to expel intestinal
worms, relieve painful
periods or bring
on menstruation.
Though, conversely, in 1652
A Directory for Midwives suggested tansy –
bruised, sprinkled with wine and applied to the navel –
to help prevent miscarriage.

Tansy is no longer taken internally, as it contains
a volatile oil which is 70 per cent thujone, potentially
damaging to the nervous system. However, pungent tansy
is an excellent insecticide and was a popular strewing
herb. Country people hung bunches of tansy flowers in
their homes and dairies to deter insects. In the days before
refrigerators, tansy was sometimes laid over (or even rubbed
into) meat to keep flies away. It is a very attractive plant,
with its fern-like leaves and yellow flowers (known as
'bitter buttons'), so it doubled as decoration in the medieval
household. A 1390 description of a Parisian wedding feast
mentioned branches of tansy decorating the table and the
bedroom. The ever-meticulous writer even told us which
market sold the best tansy, so there was obviously a thriving
trade at that time.

I grow tansy because I love its cheerful flowers and musty
scent. I press the leaves and use them in all sorts of crafts.
A friend reluctantly gave me some roots, warning that it
would spread. The Royal Horticultural Society describes
it as invasive and vigorous, and they are absolutely right.

European settlers took tansy with them to North America as a medicinal plant, and in 1638 John Josselyn reported that it was flourishing in New England gardens. It soon escaped and naturalised and has since spread everywhere. In some areas it has become a nuisance, albeit an attractive one.

∾ Skullcaps

A handsome garden plant with one-sided spires of flowers in summer is skullcap. Skullcaps (*Scutellaria* spp) get their name from the pouch on the calyx when in fruit, which does look like a shallow dish (Latin *scutella*) or a skullcap. The flowers suggested the alternative name of 'quaker's bonnet'. It is a large genus of three hundred or more species worldwide, about ninety of which are native to North America. The beautiful blue-flowered Virginian skullcap (*Scutellaria lateriflora*), in particular, which grows in marshy places all over the United States, has a reputation as a powerful treatment for nervous disorders, anxiety, depression and even St Vitus's dance. It does contain the sedative scutellarin. Scientific investigations are difficult, not least because it would be unethical to run tests on seriously anxious or depressed patients; but trials in healthy patients suggest that it does lift the mood.

The bitter leaves were thought to strengthen and stimulate the digestive system, too. The Cherokee are recorded as taking a decoction of it 'for nerves', and several tribes gave the roots of this and other *Scutellaria* species as emetics, laxatives and to hasten periods or expel afterbirth.

So not a herb to use during pregnancy. In the late eighteenth century, several New England doctors claimed great success in treating rabies with Virginian skullcap. It still has the alternative name of 'mad-dog weed', although there is no modern medical evidence to back up the claims.

The two native European skullcaps were not much written about before the late 1500s, but have also been prescribed as nervine tonics. They were reputed to have the ability to relax and stimulate at the same time. Chinese traditional medicine has long used the roots of an Asian species to combat viral infections and inflammation, and as part of a combination of treatments to support cancer patients. Modern western herbalists recommend skullcap tea, alternated with oat and vervain teas, to support the nervous system after long periods of stress or anxiety. However, the dried herb is often found adulterated with plants such as the closely related wood sage, so do buy from trusted sources, if you do not grow your own.

∾ Agrimony

Agrimony (*Agrimonia eupatoria*) is a common European native with elegant, slender spikes of small yellow flowers in summer. It grows in waste places, on roadsides and dry grassland. One of its country names is 'church spire' and another is 'cockle-bur', from the fruits which are fringed with hooks. The ancient Greeks nicknamed agrimony and similar plants *philanthropos*, 'man-loving', because the fruits stuck to their clothes. The Romans crushed agrimony with plantain and millefolium (yarrow) in wine to heal sores, and

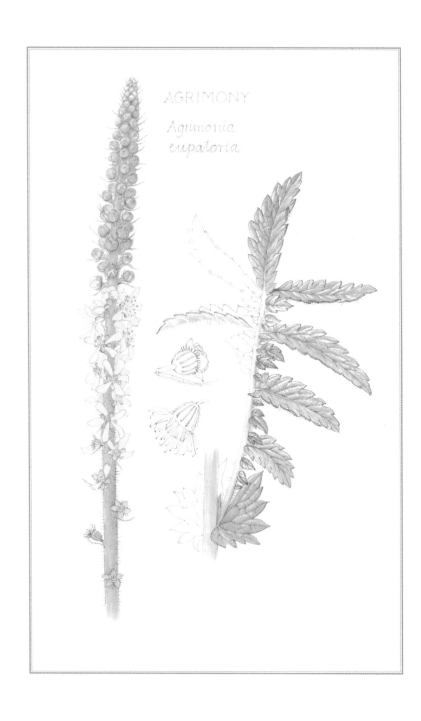

AGRIMONY

Agrimonia
eupatoria

the Anglo-Saxons gave an agrimony decoction as a wash for bleary eyes. Several herbals recommended it as a digestive tonic, and as a treatment for disorders of the gall bladder, as well as what one writer charmingly calls 'them that have naughty livers'. It is rich in tannins, which help to dry up infections, so it was prescribed to treat peptic ulcers, as well as external lesions and as a gargle for sore throats. A present-day French herbal advises gargling with a decoction of agrimony leaves and flowers twice a day for laryngitis.

But its main virtue was in stopping bleeding and treating cuts and gashes, especially battlefield wounds. Banckes's 1525 *Herbal* says agrimony is good 'to heal a wound that is hurt with iron', following traditional advice stretching back at least to Dioscorides. For thousands of years, traditional Chinese healers applied agrimony as a styptic herb, too, and recent Chinese research suggests that it does increase coagulation by up to 50 per cent.

There are two very similar-looking species in Britain, plus a third which looks quite different. The two species with tall spires of flowers, agrimony and fragrant agrimony (*Agrimonia procera*), have been seen as more or less interchangeable in folk medicine. I love the leaves of both, with their boldly toothed leaflets and flamboyant stipules. Fragrant agrimony is slightly less common, often found in damper habitats than its cousin. Its leaves smell like balsam when crushed and do make a lovely tea, reputedly an excellent tonic. In both species, the whole plant is fragrant and they have been used as strewing herbs and, more recently, in scented sachets and potpourri. Apparently, even their roots smell good, and retain their fragrance when dried.

∾ Alchemilla and parsley-piert

ALCHEMILLA

In the late 1500s, alchemilla grew wild in
many locations around London and the
south-east, but nowadays in Britain it is
almost exclusively a northern wild plant.
There are around three hundred species, most
of them originating in Europe and Asia, but some are native to
the Andes or to mountains in Africa. Several species are native
to Britain, most of them very rare and distinguished from
one another only by small details. When illustrating them
for a field guide, I had to take note of the precise number and
shape of the tiny teeth around the leaf edges and the density
of hairs on their surface. These species are generally grouped
together as the Alchemilla vulgaris aggregation.

The lovely garden plant Alchemilla mollis, originally from
the Caucasus, is widely grown and naturalised everywhere
now. It is justifiably popular as, like all its relatives, it has
frothy heads of tiny yellow, star-shaped flowers and large,
soft green leaves which hold the dew 'in drops like pearls',
as John Parkinson wrote in 1640. Dew was believed to be a
magical substance, valuable in the alchemists' quest to turn
base metal into gold. The name 'alchemilla' was coined in the
late Middle Ages to reflect this idea. Such dark magic had to
be Christianised of course, so alchemilla became known as
'lady's mantle' (i.e. Our Lady's).

Quite apart from its supposed magical properties,
alchemilla was astringent and, as Culpeper put it, 'very

proper for those wounds that have inflammation'. He said it was 'one of the most useful wound-herbs'. Poultices were applied to wounds, infusions were given to treat heavy menstruation and a decoction added to the bath was thought to prevent miscarriage. Young leaves can be added to salads, while the juice reputedly helps to clear acne. A rather startling usage, suggested in 1542 by a German physician and repeated by other writers, was in reducing and firming maidens' breasts 'when they be too great and flaggie'.

PARSLEY-PIERT

A diminutive cousin of alchemilla, the European native parsley-piert (*Aphanes arvensis*) grows in fields and on waste ground throughout Britain.
It breaks through
stony ground so, by
sympathetic magic,
was thought to break
up kidney stones and
gravel. The Normans
called it (and several
other plants) *perce-pierre*
meaning 'pierce-
stone', but its deeply
indented, slightly
frilly leaves suggested
the anglicisation
parsley-piert.

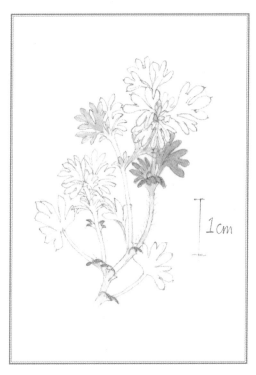

❧ Lavender

There was a big lavender bush in the front garden of the house where I was born. We brushed by it on the way to the gate, and I can remember liking the smell, even as a toddler. Every year we made lavender bags with the dried flowers, to perfume the wardrobe and linen cupboard, and to keep the moths away. Lavender has always been valued because of its strong aroma. Its name derives from the Latin *lavare*, 'to wash', as people added it to water to perfume both the body and the laundry. It was a popular strewing herb, and for centuries bags containing dried flowers or wool sprinkled with lavender oil were hung up as room fresheners and fly deterrents. Scientific research confirms its insecticidal properties: lavender oil mixed with tea-tree oil was far more effective at killing headlice than the standard treatment.

Lavenders come from the Mediterranean, North Africa, Arabia and India, but are widely cultivated everywhere now. Their natural habitat is sunny, dry, even parched rocky places. English lavender (*Lavandula angustifolia*) and its many cultivars are frost hardy to -10 °C, so thrive in temperate regions. It even escapes and naturalises occasionally – more frequently now, perhaps in response to milder winters. It is a magnet for bees, and the Roman poet Virgil recommended putting hives among bushes of lavender and thyme for the best honey.

Oil is distilled from the flowers of several lavender species, though English lavender is the one used most often. Lavender oil has a calming, soothing effect, not simply because it is pleasant. It affects the central nervous system via olfactory nerves which link directly to parts of the brain controlling emotions, so many find it to be an effective treatment for anxiety, agitation, insomnia and even post-traumatic stress disorder (PTSD). Even a bag of dried lavender flowers added to a bath would soothe nervous disorders, as well as rheumatism, according to traditional Russian folk medicine.

Clinical trials have demonstrated lavender's analgesic properties, confirming its reputation for helping with pain, especially nervous headaches. A 1485 German herbal says a small bag containing dried lavender, rose petals, bay leaves, cloves, betony and marjoram 'will soothe all pains'. It sounds delightful. Historically, lavender water was dabbed onto the temples and forehead for headaches. In addition, animal and human studies suggest that the linalool contained in lavender oil has sedative effects and can act as a depressant of the central nervous system. And an English 1790 household book gives a recipe for lavender water with the comment 'How easy it is to smell sweet.'

Lavender essential oil can be applied neat as first aid for bites, stings and burns, though it is usually diluted in a carrier oil for massage and aromatherapy.

Lavender hand balm

First I make an infused oil with dried lavender flowerheads. (This is different from the distilled oil described above.)

Put six to eight dried flowerheads into a jar, top up with a light vegetable oil, and put on a tight-fitting lid.

Gently heat the jar in a bain-marie (or a pan of simmering water) for 2 hours.

Strain and repeat the process, using new dried lavender in the same oil. Strain again.

When the oil is ready, I warm it together with beeswax — in a ratio of 4 parts oil to 1 part beeswax — in a heatproof jug set in a pan of gently simmering water.

Once the beeswax has melted, I pour the mixture into clean jars and allow to cool.

If I haven't got the consistency quite right, I simply melt it again and add more oil or wax.

The balm always cools with a dimple in the middle, so I reserve a little extra to melt and top up the jars.

It has a strong antibacterial action and was used successfully for skin wounds during the First World War. The distilled oil should not be taken internally, except under medical supervision – modern and historical writers have all urged caution. Infusions of dried flowers were prescribed for laryngitis, flu and asthma, and in a 1757 diary, the writer suggested adding lavender to flavour bitter medicines. It was sometimes included in culinary recipes, but is rather strong for the modern taste. I put a dried lavender flowerhead into a canister of sugar and then use the sugar in baking, and that is enough flavour for me. But I still hang lavender bags in the wardrobe, and a lavender pillow helps me to sleep. And the lavender hand balm opposite is a great favourite with my gardening friends.

∾ Hops

The one thing everyone knows about hops is that they are used in making beer. But it wasn't always so. Our forebears have always made a fermented ale – a safer drink than water – and flavoured it with a variety of wild plants. Bog myrtle, for instance, or yarrow or ground ivy, whose other name was 'alehoof'. Hops (Humulus lupulus) are native in temperate regions from North America and Europe to China, and no doubt some households gathered wild hop fruits to flavour their own home-made ale. There are records of hop cultivation for brewing from as early as the ninth century in and around Germany, and by the end of the Middle Ages Britain had begun to follow suit.

However, this was not without controversy: in Henry VIII's time, protestors petitioned Parliament to ban the use of hops, as they were 'a wicked weed that would spoil the taste of the drink and endanger the people'. But hops continued to grow in popularity, and soon the drink flavoured with them acquired the Germanic term 'beer', while that flavoured with other plants kept the name 'ale'. Some argued that beer was more wholesome than ale, as the hops made it a drink to keep the body healthy, rather than just to quench the thirst. As well as the medicinal benefits hops brought to beer, it was believed that they improved its keeping quality, too.

Hops have always had a reputation as a treatment for digestive and liver troubles, and for insomnia. The part used is the fruit, the papery cones – technically called 'strobiles' – which are found on female plants. Male plants have sprays of small, pale flowers instead. The fruits deteriorate quickly, so should be dried straight after picking. They should still be green, and will have a powerful smell. Country people took infusions of the fruits or plant tops to relax the digestive tract. Some herbalists made an infusion of hop fruits and chamomile as a painkilling fomentation to bathe swellings, painful joints, boils and 'gatherings'.

By far the best known medical benefit of hops is as a sedative. Clinical trials on commercial insomnia remedies containing hops, along with other ingredients such as valerian, are encouraging, though their sedative effect may be too strong for safe use by people with depression. A Russian folk remedy for insomnia advised a handful of hops under the pillow – and painting the bedroom black. The British drank infusions or, more often, sewed dried hops into a pillow. Hop pillows suddenly became very popular in the late eighteenth century, when news spread that they had cured King George III's chronic insomnia. I discovered how soporific the smell of hops can be when taking a sack-load to a friend who was making pillows for a charity sale. I found myself nodding off at the wheel and had to drive with all the windows open, while singing loudly.

When the 'country look' was all the rage, no kitchen was complete without swags of dried hop vines. The cones are smaller on wild hops than on cultivated varieties, but both are equally potent and both can cause skin irritation when handled. Hops need rich soil, and until the early twentieth century the Kent hop gardens were heavily mulched in winter with manure from London's stables. Eastenders decamped from London to the hop gardens annually in late September to harvest the fruits. Although it was hard work, the pickers partied, too. However, many of the women pickers found that their periods stopped as a result of the oestrogenic properties of hops. Over-the-counter remedies for menopausal hot flushes often contain hop extract for the same reason, and the use of hop extract in pregnancy is not recommended.

Hops are common in the wild on moist soils, often as a relic of cultivation, and cultivars with golden leaves are popular with gardeners. Hops will grow quickly and can smother other plants, hence their species name *lupulus*. This means 'little wolf', from the old nickname 'willow-wolf', referring to hops' habit of climbing over willow trees.

∾ Mugwort and its relatives

By late summer, mugwort (*Artemisia vulgaris*) is flourishing on roadsides, field margins and waste ground everywhere. It is tall and bushy, but so common we hardly notice it, considering it a weed. A friend's father, brought up on a Surrey farm in the 1920s, knew it as 'dungweed', because it always grew on the dung heap. Scholars debate about whether it was called 'mugwort' because it was used to flavour the beer in your mug, or from an old word for maggot, because it would keep the moth larvae out of your wardrobe. It was so easily available in the wild that it was rarely cultivated, except in a few physic gardens. Healers would collect the leaves in August, and dig the roots in autumn to dry.

Dioscorides called it 'artemisia' and prescribed it for gynaecological troubles. An infusion of the flowers taken as a drink, or a sitz bath with a decoction of leaves in it, would help to bring on periods, hasten expulsion of the afterbirth and heal inflammations of the womb, as well as break down kidney stones. A poultice of the leaves, mixed with myrrh and applied externally to the lower abdomen, would have similar effects. There are reports of Chinese and Siberian folk healers

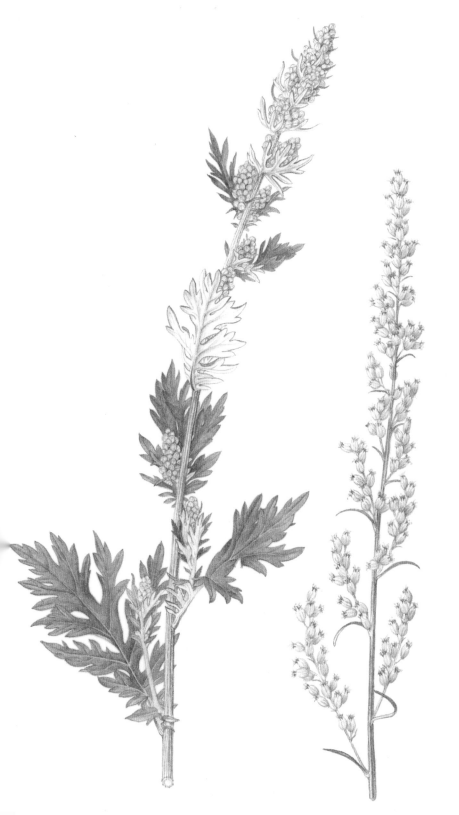

using mugwort root for the same conditions. An English seventeenth-century household book advised an infusion of mugwort and cloves in wine 'for a poor country woman in labour to hasten her birth'. Please don't try any of this at home!

Mugwort was a favourite herb with the Anglo-Saxons, who prescribed it for the treatment of kidney stones and strangury, painful joints, carbuncles and skin sores, as well as 'women's troubles'. In traditional Chinese medicine, the pale down was scraped from the underside of the leaves and pressed into 'moxa' cones, which were burnt on the skin to relieve rheumatism and arthritis. In seventeenth-century Britain, the use of daisies to treat bruises, lumps and wens was said to be more effective with the addition of mugwort.

Another plant closely related to mugwort is wormwood (Artemisia absinthium), which, as its name suggests, was a vermifuge. It was also used to flavour the notorious drink absinthe, which, taken in excess, caused hallucinations and delirium due to the thujone in the herb. Mugwort also contains thujone, and has been used in attempts to induce lucid, or at least vivid, dreams. Although mugwort is recommended in some modern herbals for digestive and menstruation problems, it should only be taken under the guidance of a qualified expert.

There are many related Artemisia species (sagebrushes and wormwoods) in North America. The Navajo, Paiute and many others gave them for coughs and colds, fevers, sores and sprains, but also to provoke abortions. So artemisias are definitely herbs to be avoided during pregnancy. But on the positive side, the Shoshoni and others made sagebrush decoctions to relieve pain after childbirth.

Mugwort was another of the 'flowers of St John', traditionally blessed in the smoke of midsummer fires and hung in the house for protection from evil. Gerard would have none of its assumed magical properties. Such 'fantastical devices', he wrote, were 'tending to witchcraft and sourcery'. He would omit them as 'things unworthy of my recording or your reviewing'. Though he couldn't resist repeating Dioscorides' claim that putting mugwort in your shoes would prevent you from tiring on long journeys.

∾ Vervain

Common vervain (*Verbena officinalis*) – also called 'common verbena' – grows wild on dry, calcareous soils throughout most of Europe, apart from in the extreme north. Gardeners have cultivated it since at least medieval times, and it has now escaped into the wild everywhere. Many colourful hybrids have been bred from related *Verbena* species for our gardens, but wild vervain itself is rather spindly, with dark, pinnate leaves and thin spikes of pale-lilac flowers.

Classical authors referred to it as *hiera botane*, the 'sacred plant', valuable in purification ceremonies in temples and homes. It was not just the Romans who believed vervain to have magical powers. The Gauls, wrote Pliny, used it in prophesying, and their Magi (druids) made 'the maddest statements' about the plant. It was another of the midsummer protective plants, later Christianised as 'herbs of St John' or the 'holy herb'.

The name 'vervain' comes from the Celtic words *fer* 'to chase away' and *faen* 'stone'. Pliny says it is 'a sovereign remedy for stone' and gives a very long list of other conditions it would help, including scrofula, epilepsy, dysentery, swollen parotid glands, dropsy, jaundice, gout, chronic ulcers and even corns and 'sores caused by footwear'. Chewing a root would strengthen the gums and teeth, or a decoction in wine or vinegar could be used as a mouthwash. A decoction of the root would treat troubles at or after childbirth. The tenth-century *Lacnunga* says that vervain was good for those 'sore of liver', among other things.

In medieval Europe, vervain was famous as a headache remedy. A 1507 German herbal claimed that wearing a vervain garland round the head night and day for a headache 'helps wonderfully'. More usually, the aerial parts were made into an infusion and drunk. Physicians valued vervain greatly, but it did gather many 'old wives' tales' which a few writers reported and most rejected. Recently, vervain has become popular as a treatment for stress-related headaches, migraine and nervous exhaustion, as well as for the liver and gall bladder – though doctors warn that taking too large a dose for too long can be dangerous, and it should be avoided in pregnancy. A modern French herbal advises pouring 250ml (8.7fl oz) of boiling water onto a small handful of vervain and allowing it to infuse for 10 minutes, before straining and drinking for headaches, but take expert advice to be sure you are taking a safe and appropriate dose.

❧ Valerian

Another well-known herbal treatment for the nervous system is valerian. Not the popular red valerian (*Centranthus ruber*), which spills clouds of red (or white) flowers and fleshy glaucous leaves over summer garden walls. I mean the European native common valerian (*Valeriana officinalis*) – a tall, more delicate plant with dark, pinnate leaves and fragrant heads of small, pale flowers. It grows in damp places and rough grassland throughout most of Europe and has been grown in herb gardens for centuries. The name 'valerian' first appears in eleventh-century herbal recipes, but Chaucer knew it as 'setwall' and others as 'all-heal'.

The rather pungent root was a powerful sedative, used in treatments for headache, nervous exhaustion and stress-related digestive disorders. It was also reputed to strengthen the heart, and tests have shown that it may indeed reduce blood pressure.

In Italy, in 1592, Fabius Calumna claimed that valerian root had cured his epilepsy, and from then on European physicians prescribed it for that and

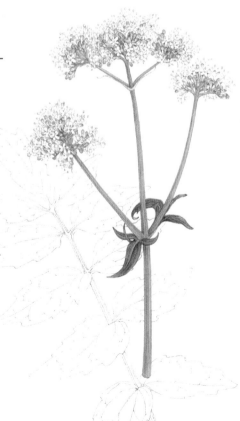

for conditions like St Vitus's dance and vertigo. In Canada, the Woodland Cree nation made woods valerian (*Valeriana dioica* var. *sylvatica*) into a poultice applied externally for seizures in infants. A Himalayan species is used in Ayurvedic medicine for insomnia and nervous disorders. In Europe, valerian has a long, unofficial history of successfully treating melancholy (depression), anxiety, insomnia and menopausal hot flushes. However, research suggests that, if taken over a long period (more than four to six weeks), there could be withdrawal issues. In France, the sale of valerian is restricted.

Physicians down the ages have valued valerian highly for its medicinal virtues, and it is still sold in commercial preparations today. It is a sedative, so never use it when driving, as large doses are said to 'stupefy'.

Golden rod

In the garden of the house where I grew up there was a huge clump of golden rod, which flowered late in the summer. My mother was allergic to the pollen and spent most of September sneezing. This was a tall garden variety of golden rod (*Solidago canadensis*), which, as its name suggests, comes from North America, like most species in the genus. It was introduced to Europe in 1648. The flowers, like little golden shaving brushes, are crowded together along arching racemes. It is always popular with pollinators. Like some other introduced plants, it is rather invasive, spreading both by root and by seeds. Gardeners have often thrown it out, only for it to establish itself in the wild, becoming a common wasteland weed. In

North America, the Iroquois used it as an emetic; the Syilx to stop diarrhoea; and the Zuni to treat sore throats and coughs. Infusions or decoctions of other American species were applied as washes to heal wounds, burns and sores, or drunk for fevers.

In Britain, we treated the same range of conditions with Europe's own native golden rod (*Solidago virgaurea*). A smaller plant than its American cousins, it has flowers with ray florets, as well as disc florets – like small yellow daisies. *Solidago* comes from the Latin *solidus*, meaning 'whole', as it would make wounds and sores whole again. Herbalists sang its praises as a wound herb, stopping bleeding in any part of the body, including the 'bloody flux' (dysentery) and 'immoderate women's courses'. Golden rod was (and is) best known as an effective diuretic treatment for stones and kidney infections, too. There is a 1788 record of a ten-year-old boy, treated for some time with infusions of golden rod, passing an eye-watering number of sizeable stones, poor lad. Modern scientific research confirms that golden rod is effective in treating some chronic bladder conditions, reducing pain and urgency. Plenty of other fluids should be taken alongside infusions of the flowering tops.

Gerard thought very highly of golden rod and noted how the imported dried herb had once cost half a crown an ounce, but when it was found growing abundantly in Hampstead woods, on the edge of London, no one would pay half a crown a hundredweight. He complained at length that people, especially 'fantastical Physicians', only valued herbs that were 'strange and rare'. He pointed out to these 'new fangled fellows' that golden rod had just the same virtues now that it was common, as it had had when it was thought to be rare.

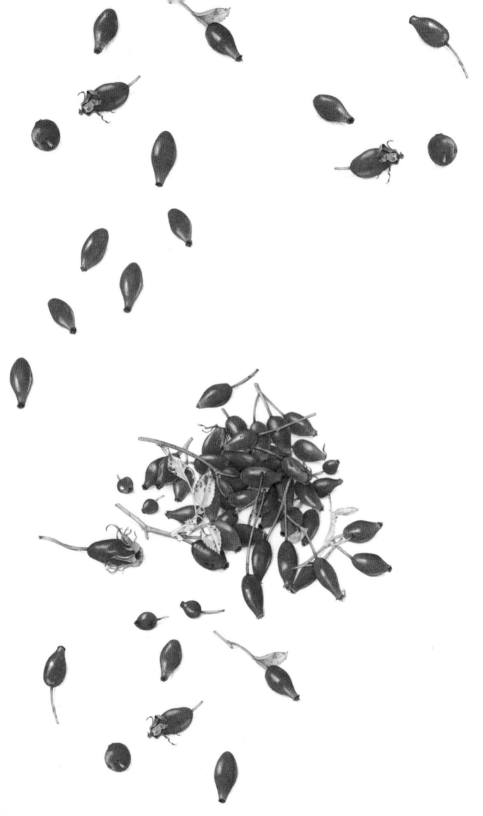

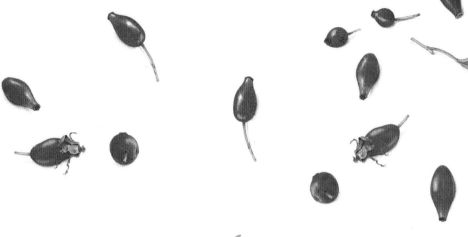

Autumn

The teeming autumn, big with rich increase

WILLIAM SHAKESPEARE,
'Sonnet 97' (1609)

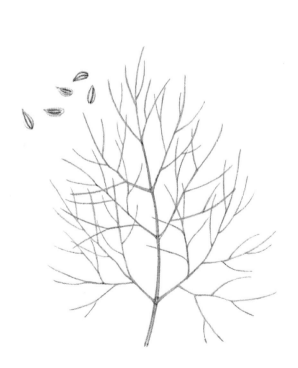

As summer ripens into autumn, the fields and hedgerows provide an abundance of fruits and berries too tempting to ignore – a free source of food, and of medicine, too. Early autumn has always been the time for collecting seeds, to plant in spring for next year's harvest, to add flavour in cooking or to make useful remedies.

The roots of some plants were also medicinally valuable, often having different properties to the aerial parts. Theophrastus wrote that most roots were dug in autumn 'after the rising of Arcturus, when the plants have shed their leaves'. Most writers gave advice on cleaning and drying roots. They sensibly advised checking once a month to ensure that the roots hadn't gone soft. Properly dried roots would last up to a year, they said. Some families would have dug roots for their own use, but physicians and apothecaries were supplied by professional 'herb-diggers' up until the twentieth century. In Elizabethan England, the Wild Herb Act confirmed the diggers' rights to collect in wild or uncultivated places, such as lane sides and field edges. This is no longer legal.

∾ Raspberry leaf

Raspberry (Rubus idaeus) is native in open woodlands and downland over most of Europe and, of course, is widely

cultivated everywhere. Its
red fruits ripen in summer
or early autumn, and there are
some easy-care garden varieties that
fruit in late autumn. Its old name
was 'hindberry', 'raspberry' being
first recorded in 1532. Dioscorides
referred to it as 'Idean bramble',
the bramble from Mount Ida, and
Linnaeus preserved this connection when
he gave it its scientific name. Although a member of the rose
family, instead of producing big berries or hips each with
lots of seeds inside, its fruits are composed of a collection
of 'drupelets', each containing a single seed. All its *Rubus*
relatives do the same, and you can often see the dried-up
remains of the stigma attached to each drupelet.

The Romans recommended infusions of raspberry flowers
for skin conditions, sore eyes and digestive disorders. The
berries were considered very nourishing and do, in fact,
contain vitamins A, B, C and E, as well as iron, calcium and
phosphorus. An infusion of dried raspberry leaves was given
as a gargle, or for diarrhoea and fevers in children. An Anglo-
Saxon manuscript includes *hindbergean* (raspberries) in several
remedies for lung disease. But its best-known use was as a
birth aid, taken in the last weeks of pregnancy.

In many parts of Europe, the favourite medication for
pregnant women hoping for a swift and easy birth has always
been raspberry-leaf tea, an infusion made with dried leaves.
There is a very long-standing and widespread tradition of
its use in unofficial country medicine. Recent clinical trials

have shown no significant benefit, but found no adverse side effects either – though, as with all herbs, never use during pregnancy without taking medical advice first. Some midwives and doctors insist that it really does help – so the jury is (as they say) still out.

∽ Blackberry or bramble

Blackberry bushes (Rubus fruticosus) are so well known that most writers agree with Culpeper that they 'need no description': they are 'every where in hedges'. They and closely related species grow wild all over Europe, Asia and North America and, since being introduced into Australia in the nineteenth century, they have become a nuisance weed there. They do grow and spread rapidly, their long stems (technically 'stolons') arching over and rooting at the tips, quickly forming an impenetrable thicket. Unsurprisingly, blackberries were not normally grown in gardens until the late eighteenth century, when thornless, ornamental or (hopefully) better-behaved varieties were developed. Blackberries were abundant in the wild – Shakespeare even used the simile 'as plentiful as blackberries'. Growing up, we went out blackberrying every year, gathering delicious, free berries from every hedgerow. Buying blackberries in expensive punnets in the supermarket just isn't the same.

The names 'blackberry' and 'bramble' come down to us virtually unchanged from the Anglo-Saxons, and the scientific name Rubus is simply what the Romans called it. In fact, like the dandelion, blackberry is not a single species, but an aggregation of many micro-species – over 320 in the British Isles alone … and counting. Despite the slight differences, their flowers all attract a multitude of butterflies and other insects, and their fruit is important to a wide range of wildlife – and, of course, to us. A well-preserved Neolithic man excavated in Essex in 1911 was found to have blackberry seeds in his stomach. As well as eating the fruit, our ancestors made twine out of the fibrous stems, collected the sheep's wool caught on the prickles and used various parts of the plant for dyes. The roots gave an orange tint; the fruits a range of pinks, purples and slate greys; and, as writers since Dioscorides have reported, the leaves could dye your hair black, while at the same time healing an itchy or infected scalp.

The tannins which made brambles so useful in dyeing also meant that they made excellent styptic medicines, drying up both external and internal conditions. Pliny and Dioscorides both recommended chewing the leaves to clear up mouth ulcers and strengthen the gums, and applying poultices of leaves to heal skin sores – though both said that including bruised stalks as well worked even better. In 1771, John Cruso's *Treasure of Easy Medicine* advised a decoction of leaves for persistent skin ulcers, and there are records of nineteenth-century country people from the Scottish Highlands to Cornwall applying bramble leaves to swellings, septic wounds and burns. Early twentieth-century Dorset folk made bramble tips and primroses into an ointment to heal spots and sores on the face.

Closely related *Rubus* species growing elsewhere were just as astringent. In North America, the Iroquois,

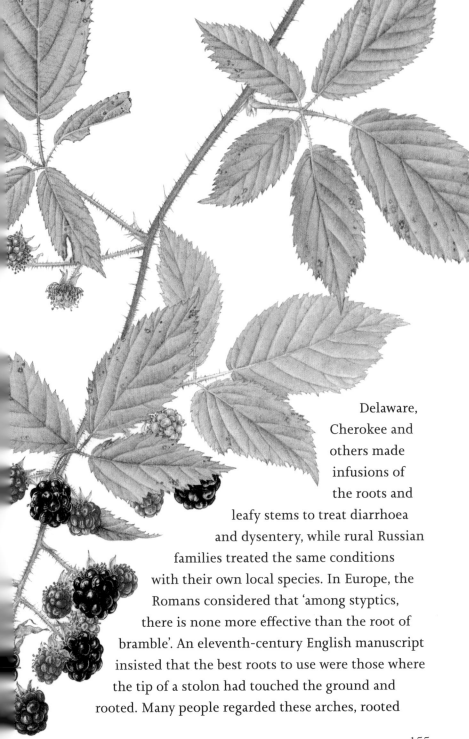

Delaware,
Cherokee and
others made
infusions of
the roots and
leafy stems to treat diarrhoea
and dysentery, while rural Russian
families treated the same conditions
with their own local species. In Europe, the
Romans considered that 'among styptics,
there is none more effective than the root of
bramble'. An eleventh-century English manuscript
insisted that the best roots to use were those where
the tip of a stolon had touched the ground and
rooted. Many people regarded these arches, rooted

at both ends, as magical, and believed that passing a child through the arch would cure 'chincough' (whooping cough). They said the same about rheumatism, though expecting someone with painful joints to crawl through a low, prickly hoop is asking a lot.

People have always enjoyed related species, such as dewberry (*Rubus caesius*), whose fruits consist of fewer, bigger drupelets covered with a white, waxy bloom. A Sussex botanist, writing in about 1800, remarked what a pleasant fruit dewberries were; he went on to say that if added to red wine, they gave it a 'fine flavour'. Cloudberry (*Rubus chamaemorus*) grows in northern and upland regions around the northern hemisphere. Swedish friends relish their annual outings to harvest its orange berries. To be honest, I don't find they taste of much; but in latitudes with very short summers, they are a welcome free source of vitamin C. Both dewberry and cloudberry have been used in country medicine in the same ways as blackberry.

The familiar blackberry has the highest vitamin A content of any berry fruit, so it is well worth picking to eat, freeze or cook. I sometimes make blackberries (and raspberries) into syrups or vinegars, then dilute them in hot water as a drink or to soothe a sore throat. Several writers advise squeezing the juice from ripe blackberries into a bowl and leaving it in a warm place overnight. It will turn into a lovely, dark sauce the consistency of thick cream – not only delicious, but excellent 'mouth medicine'. The berry at the tip of the panicle ripens first, and is the sweetest, then berries further back ripen over the following weeks. There is an old superstition that blackberries should not be picked after Michaelmas Day (11 October, by the old calendar) as the Devil had spat or urinated on them. This does make sense, as late berries are often rather unpleasant, spoilt by insects and bacteria.

∾ Bilberries and their relatives

With so many similar-looking species, you will need a good identification guide when foraging in the wild.

BILBERRY, BLUEBERRY

On moorlands and in acid woodlands in Europe and north Asia, knee-high bilberry bushes produce their berries in August. Bilberry (*Vaccinium myrtillus*) often hides its blue–black berries under its leaves, so gathering a decent amount is time consuming, but well worth it for their flavour, let alone their health benefits. They are delicious! Other vernacular names are 'whortleberry', 'whinberry' and 'blaeberry'. Picking them was once a commercial activity, with whole families spending days out on the moors, 'whorting'. The harvest was sent off to be used in dyeing or for jam-making, earning the family enough to buy shoes for the winter. In France, I have enjoyed *myrtilles* (bilberries) in patisserie, preserves, a delicious and powerful liqueur and a beautiful purple ice cream.

Bilberries were highly thought of by the ancients, and have been used for centuries as a home remedy for diarrhoea. The leaves had a reputation for helping in diabetes, and the berries for strengthening the cardiovascular system and improving retinal conditions in the eye. Clinical research in all three areas shows encouraging results, and the anthocyanin in bilberries makes them an excellent antioxidant, too. Bilberries were historically also prescribed for fevers, coughs and urinary tract infections. Efforts made in the nineteenth century to cultivate them were abandoned with the introduction of their larger (and less flavoursome) American cousin, the blueberry. Today's commercially grown blueberries come from hybrids between two species native to North America. Blueberries have similar health benefits to bilberries – but, to me, a blueberry tart cannot compete with a *tarte aux myrtilles* for flavour.

From the top: bilberry fruit and flower; blueberry; cowberry; bearberry; American cranberry; European cranberry.

COWBERRY

A close relative of the bilberry, and growing in similar habitats all over Eurasia and North America, is cowberry (*Vaccinium vitis-idaea*). Also known as 'lingonberry' and 'partridge-berry', its shiny red berries were eaten by the Tanana people of Alaska to treat coughs and colds. In the Middle Ages in Britain they were given for diarrhoea. Gerard reported that he himself had used cowberry juice for 'limning' (painting), and that it made a perfect 'carnation' (flesh colour). Cowberries are safe to eat, but are very tart, so its relatives might be preferable – remedies might as well taste good!

CRANBERRY

The European cranberry (*Vaccinium oxycoccus*), another closely related plant found in northern, central and eastern Europe, is a creeping plant with tiny, widely spaced leaves and small red fruits. It grows in acid bogs in Britain, where it is widespread only in the north and west. The American cranberry (*Vaccinium macrocarpon*), with its bigger fruits, provides the cranberries we eat with our roast turkey at Christmas or Thanksgiving. This species has been cultivated since the early eighteenth century, though with difficulty. A breeding programme in the 1920s required a sort of artificial bog on which cranberry's creeping stems formed a mat in the first year, then more upright shoots in the second year and flowers and fruit in the third year. However, harvesting the berries was tricky and there was a good deal of wastage.

159

The Innu nation in eastern Canada made an infusion of cranberry branches to treat pleurisy, and others used it for digestive disorders and to purify the blood. Today, cranberry juice is celebrated as a treatment for cystitis. Despite a great deal of anecdotal evidence, the many clinical trials have failed to prove any significant benefits for this condition. However, it was discovered that cranberry boosts the immune system and, while test patients did not avoid catching colds or flu altogether, they suffered fewer symptoms. Cranberry juice contains a lot of natural sugars, so people with diabetes should perhaps look for a sugar-free alternative.

BEARBERRY

A slightly more distant relative that is also credited with alleviating cystitis is bearberry (*Arctostaphylos uva-ursi*), which grows on stony or peaty soil in northern regions around the globe, and on mountains further south. If you prefer to grow bearberry in your garden, you can hasten germination of the ripe seeds by soaking them in boiling water for 15 seconds before planting. Bearberry is well named – or at least thoroughly named: *Arctostaphylos* is from the Greek for 'bear grape' and *uva-ursi* means the same in Latin, echoing its English name – all from the belief that bears like to eat the scarlet berries.

Bearberry's leathery leaves were made into a diuretic decoction given for urinary tract disorders such as gravel, ulcers and cystitis. Everyone used bearberry this way, from the 'Physicians of Myddfai' in twelfth-century Wales to the Cheyenne and Cherokee in North America. In the 1930s, the official British Pharmacopoeia advised that the leaves should be collected in September or October and dried in the shade. They do contain a good percentage of arbutin, which the body converts into hydroquinone, soothing and disinfecting the urinary tract. Too much hydroquinone can be dangerous, so bearberry should not be taken long term. As it is hard to distinguish the leaves from other plants, it might be wise to use a commercial preparation, just to be sure of identification and correct dosage. Clinical trials do show bearberry to be effective in mild cystitis; but if you have a fever, pain or blood in the urine, you should get medical help urgently.

∾ Rose hips

Probably the most noticeable autumn fruits in the hedgerow and garden are glossy, scarlet rose hips. Botanically speaking, they are 'false fruits', actually the swollen receptacle, the end of the flower stalk. Often you can see the colour bleeding a little way into the stem – there is no sharp division. The actual fruit is the fibrous down inside, surrounding the hard, yellow seeds. This 'rough cotton', as it was known, is an irritant, used by generations of children as 'itching powder'. Wild rose flowers were not much valued in medicine, and the cultivated varieties were preferred. Gerard grew several wild roses in his London garden, but drew the line at the dog rose (Rosa canina) as being unworthy. It was common enough in the wild. He listed several places where it grew in abundance, including a path 'from a village hard by London called Knight's Bridge, unto Fulham, a village thereby'. I doubt there are many dog roses to be found between Knightsbridge and Fulham nowadays.

All rose hips are edible, but when foraging, do make sure that the bushes have not been sprayed with chemicals. In Britain, the dog rose, or 'hep-bush', was the best source of hips, which Tudor 'cooks and gentlewomen' made into tarts and other sweet dishes. The flavour is sharp and sweet at the same time. The hips of other species were used, too, and all had to have the insides either scraped out before cooking or strained out afterwards to avoid irritating the digestive tract. Rose hips have been eaten for a very long time – they have been discovered at Neolithic sites. The Romans advised an infusion of rose hips to check diarrhoea

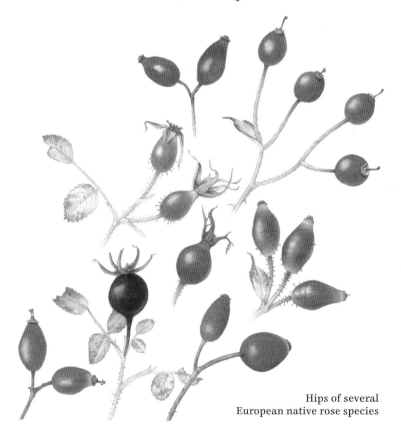

Hips of several
European native rose species

and haemorrhage, and in 1652 Culpeper wrote that rose hip conserve, made with sugar, was a digestive treatment 'besides the pleasantness of the taste'. In Russian folk medicine, a hawthorn infusion given for angina also included rose hips for sweetness. Modern clinical trials with powdered rose hip preparations indicate that they have an anti-inflammatory effect, significantly reducing pain in osteoarthritis.

Rose hips contain an extraordinary amount of vitamin C – around twenty times as much as an orange – and this fact led to its most famous application in wartime Britain. With the importation of citrus fruits halted, the Ministry of Health was concerned that people – children especially – could suffer vitamin deficiency. In 1941, the collection of rose hips from the wild to make National Rose Hip Syrup began. Schools, church halls and community buildings became collection points, and collectors were paid 3d for a pound of hips. Burnet rose (*Rosa spinosissima*), the only British native rose with black hips, contains even more vitamin C, so commanded 4d a pound. The County Herb Committees oversaw the collection, which by the end of the war was around an impressive 450 tons each year. The syrup was sold at a fixed price to families with small children. It is still marketed today, now made from wild roses cultivated specially. Many country people made their own, and some of us still do. It is delicious drizzled over ice cream, or diluted as a hot cordial, which was also reputed to ward off colds and flu. A small study showed that a commercial rose hip drink helped restore 'good' bacteria to the gut, which is a bonus. There are many recipes for rose hip syrup; the one below is adapted from a mid-twentieth-century Women's Institute recipe.

Rose hip syrup

For every 500g of rose hips, I use 1.5 litres of water and 225g of sugar.

(Or 1 lb hips, 2¼ pints water and ½ lb sugar.)

Put two thirds of the water (850ml, 1½ pints) into a large pan and bring it to the boil. One writer says that using an enamel pan will preserve the lovely rosy colour. Wash the hips, remove any stalks and dried sepals, then mince or chop them finely in the food processor and add them to the pan of boiling water. Bring back to the boil, remove from the heat and allow to stand for about 15 minutes.

Pour into a jelly bag and allow the juice to drip through into a large bowl. Don't be tempted to squeeze the bag, or those irritant little hairs may get through.

Put the remaining water into the pan and bring it to the boil. When all the liquid has dripped through the jelly bag, empty the rose hip pulp back into the pan. Bring it back to the boil, remove from the heat, and allow to stand for 10 minutes or so. Pour into a clean jelly bag set over the bowl containing the first lot of juice.

Pour the juice into a clean pan and boil until reduced to 425ml (¾ pint). (I find a good way of checking this is to practise beforehand with 425ml (¾ pint) water in the pan and mark the level on a wooden skewer.) Add the sugar and stir until completely dissolved. Pour into sterilised bottles and seal, or cool and pour into freezer containers. Small bottles or containers are best, as this syrup only keeps for a week or so once opened.

❧ Mustard seed

As autumn progresses, other plants start to produce their
seeds. A path I often walk along is lined with black mustard
plants (*Brassica nigra*), almost as tall as I am. In the spring,
I forage its young leaves for salads; but in the autumn,
I collect some of its pods. They are held upright against the
stem and are smooth, with a small pointed beak. The small
seeds are dark-brown or black. If I can find white mustard
(*Sinapis alba*), I collect its pods, too. They have a long flat beak
at the end and are held away from the main stem. Its yellow
seeds are bigger and milder. I leave plenty of pods behind, as
both species are annual, growing from seed each year.

Excavations at Neolithic villages have found evidence of
a surprisingly varied range of foodstuffs, including mustard.
Originally native to Europe, mustards are widely cultivated
around the world and often escape into the wild, though
there are several similar yellow-flowered relatives, such as
charlock or rape. The yellow mustard fields of 1950s Britain
have given way to fields of oil-seed rape, a magnet for
bees, but producing a pale, solid, odd-tasting honey. Even
the mustard-and-cress of childhood is now more likely to
include rape than mustard seeds. In 1699, John Evelyn said
mustard seedlings would 'quicken and revive the spirits,
strengthening the memory, expelling heaviness'. A good
reason for growing it on my windowsill throughout the year.

More mature mustard leaves have been – and still are –
eaten as a pot-herb wherever it grows. In ancient Greece,
Theophrastus gave a detailed description of white mustard's
cultivation, though he said that the wild kind is stronger and

more pungent. It appears in medieval garden lists, and I have seen terraced fields of it in modern-day Nepal. The seeds of both mustards have always been used to make a hot, pungent sauce which goes well with roast meat. A fourteenth-century French household-management book, listing the requirements for a wedding feast, says that forty guests would need 2 quarts (4 pints, or 2.27 litres) of mustard!

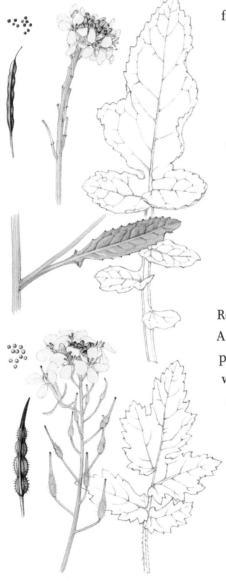

Throughout history, people have eaten mustard seeds to clear the head and lungs and to stimulate the body. Pliny advised mixing ground mustard with vinegar and using it as smelling salts to revive lethargic patients or women who had fainted. (Perhaps Roman men did not faint.) A weak solution of mustard powder would act as a laxative, while a stronger one was an emetic. An old Siberian remedy for a cold was to sprinkle dry mustard powder inside your woollen socks, while a mustard foot bath would prevent you from catching a cold in the first place. Mustard foot baths were always a popular way of stimulating the circulation, though lampooned in many old cartoons. If you have tired, aching feet, mix 2 teaspoons of mustard powder with about 2 litres (roughly 4 pints) of hot water and soak your feet for 20 minutes. If your feet are very cold, warm them gradually or you will encourage chilblains. For deep-seated conditions, mustard poultices were applied to the skin, though they often caused blisters. In fact, since classical times blistering was considered to be helpful, drawing internal illness to the surface. Modern medicine disagrees.

In medieval England, the best mustard was that grown in Tewkesbury, Gloucestershire. 'Tewkesbury mustard' even gets a mention in Shakespeare's Henry IV. Ground seed was mixed with honey or vinegar and made into balls, which kept well. Then, when you wanted some mustard, you simply moistened a ball with more vinegar. At the end of the eighteenth century, a process was invented for producing fine mustard powder using un-hulled white and black mustard seeds, sometimes with turmeric added for colour. Whenever we had roast beef, ham or sausages, mixing mustard in the blue glass pot inside its silver holder was a familiar ritual, akin to making mint sauce for roast lamb.

୬ Fennel and its relatives

Another family of plants which have given us food and medicine for centuries is the Apiaceae or Umbelliferae. A painter in one of my classes very aptly misnamed them the 'umbrellifers' as all the flower stalks arise from a single point, like the spokes of an umbrella. But it is a treacherous family, giving us tasty parsley, celery, fennel and dill, but also toxic plants like hemlock, fool's parsley and giant hogweed. So, more than ever, foragers need a good identification guide to help them correctly identify the right plant. Most of the plants described here have long been grown in herb gardens for their leaves; but, apart from British archaeophytes fennel and caraway, the seeds would not have ripened without the long, hot summers of their native lands. So the plants rarely escaped into the wild, and cooks and healers relied on imported seeds. With the climate warming, however, that could change.

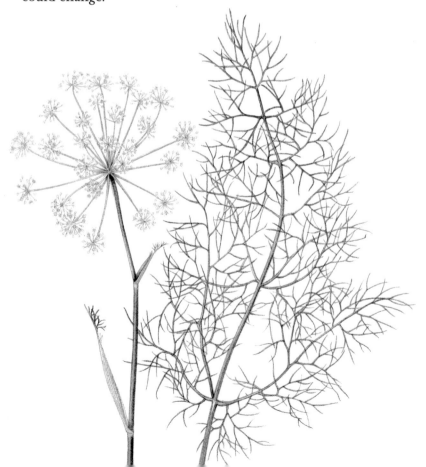

FENNEL

Fennel (*Foeniculum vulgare*) is unmistakable, with its feathery, dark-green leaves and yellow flowers. The leaflets are hair-like and not all in one plane – and they have that characteristic aniseed smell. Fennel goes well with fish dishes, and the young shoots were candied by seventeenth-century French confectioners and sold as breath fresheners. Fennel probably came to Britain in Roman times (an archaeophyte) and has naturalised happily on waste ground, as it has done around the world. Gardeners grow many types of fennel, such as Florence fennel (var. *dulce*), whose fleshy leaf-bases are a tasty vegetable, and the lovely bronze fennel (cv. Purpurascens), with clouds of deep-brown leaves. There are bronze and green fennel plants by a favourite path near my home, and I often collect a few leaves to make tea or chop into salads. I also collect the seeds in autumn.

Fennel seeds (botanically speaking, they are fruits, not seeds) were a painkiller and had the reputation of increasing the flow of milk. Hippocrates and Dioscorides both recommended it to nursing mothers, and in 1639 *The Widdowes Treasure* gave a recipe for parsnip and fennel roots in broth, which 'makes your milk increase'. Fennel, like celery, alexanders and parsley, has been prescribed ever since the ancient Greeks as a diuretic to expel bladder stones. The Anglo-Saxons considered fennel one of their 'nine sacred herbs', and it appears frequently in their leechbooks. In the twelfth century, German Abbess Hildegard of Bingen wrote that fennel 'makes a person happy ... and makes his digestion good'. I must say the smell of fennel leaves always

169

lifts my spirits. The main medicinal use of fennel, however, has always been for the digestion. Like coriander, cumin and caraway, seeds of fennel were made into a tea to settle indigestion and flatulence. It was even gentle enough to give as an infusion to babies with colic, though you should, of course, check with a health professional before introducing herbs to babies. Studies show that it does seem to help relax internal muscle. Large medicinal doses of fennel seeds should be avoided in pregnancy.

DILL

Dill (Anethum graveolens) was known in ancient Egypt, and the remains of a flowering leafy stem was found on the mummy of Amenhotep II (d. 1400 BCE). Philistion, a fourth century BCE Greek physician, advised cabbage juice in vinegar with dill, coriander, honey and pepper to cure hiccups, and dill has always been known to aid digestion. Banckes's 1525 Herbal stated that 'it assuages rumbling in a man's womb [stomach] and wicked winds in the womb. Also, it destroys the yexing [hiccups].' Like fennel, dill water or 'gripe water' was given to colicky babies, as recommended by Mrs Beeton in 1861. Dill looks like fennel, though with very slightly wider and flatter leaflets. It, too, is served with fish, and the unripe flowerheads give a distinctive taste to pickles. It is occasionally found in Britain as a casual growing on waste ground.

ANISE

Anise (*Pimpinella anisum*) was also well known to the ancient Egyptians, and in biblical times it was so highly valued that it could be used in payment: 'tithe of mint and anise and cummin' (Matthew 23:23). It is mentioned in Pharaonic medical texts as a digestive treatment, and Pliny said 'nothing is considered to be more beneficial to the belly and intestines'. This view was repeated down the ages: for example, in 1670, when Hannah Woolley advised oil of anise in sack (sherry) for 'griping of the guts'.

Pliny also suggested that the smell of anise on your pillow would help you to sleep, while its insecticidal qualities would rid you of lice, should the need arise. Anise is expectorant, so was also given for coughs, especially long-standing 'tight' coughs. A seventeenth-century household book includes anise in a complicated recipe for a 'water' to treat consumption. Although there was so much alcohol in it that 'water' doesn't seem the right term. Star anise (*Illicium verum*) has the same properties as anise, and I often pop one into a cup of boiling water for an after-dinner drink. Anise is a flavouring in liqueurs such as Pernod and ouzo, though anisette is flavoured with star anise. Since Roman days people have chewed anise to freshen their breath, a forerunner of the aniseed balls of our childhood.

CARAWAY

Excavations have revealed fossilised caraway seeds in mesolithic sites dating back at least 5,000 years, and caraway

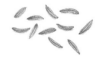

(*Carum carvi*), was known to physicians in the ancient Middle East. It has been grown in Britain's physic gardens since at least 1300 and is now naturalised in other parts of the world, too. Medieval banquets were rounded off with 'caraway comfits' to sweeten the breath and reduce any ill-effects from overindulgence. Sir Hugh Plat's *Delightes for Ladies* (1600) describes the very laborious process of making comfits by coating seeds with multiple layers of sugar syrup, while stirring them vigorously with your hand and drying them out between each coat. In the Middle Ages, fruit was always served with caraway, and in Shakespeare's *Henry IV*, Squire Shallow offers Falstaff a 'last year's pippin of my own grafting, with a dish of caraways'. Caraway seeds are often baked into bread and cakes, though not everyone appreciates the strong flavour. Like its relatives, caraway aids digestion and prevents flatulence. When stir-frying finely shredded kale or braising red cabbage in the oven, I often include a pinch of caraway seeds for their flavour and to make it more digestible. Caraway was added to medicines, too, to improve the taste and to soften the effects of harsh laxative ingredients.

CORIANDER

Another related plant with aromatic seeds credited with digestive benefits is coriander (*Coriandrum sativum*), known in America as 'cilantro'. *Sativum* means 'useful', and coriander is certainly used a great deal in cooking, especially in Middle Eastern and Asian dishes, though it is becoming popular in western cooking, too. Carrot and coriander soup is a great favourite, made with the leaves. They have a strong flavour, while the round seeds (fruits) have a gentler, more perfumed note. Coriander also comes from the eastern Mediterranean, and is occasionally found in Britain growing as a casual, especially around areas where Asian communities live.

Coriander has been a digestive aid since at least 1500 BCE and is mentioned in ancient Egyptian medical texts and in the writings of Hippocrates. In the first century CE, Pliny recommended fresh garlic and coriander in wine as both 'purgative and aphrodisiac' – not a happy combination, surely? He went on to report that a near-contemporary, scholar and satirist Marcus Terentius Varro, thought that 'by slightly pounded coriander and cumin, with vinegar, meat of any kind can be kept sweet in the heat of summer'. Coriander is in fact slightly antiseptic. The first century CE also saw the publication of a collection of food-writings attributed to Apicius. Among the recipes are several for 'Alexandrian sauce', which included coriander and cumin, and was served with fish and (for the vegetarians) marrow.

CUMIN

Cumin appears as an ingredient in many ancient Egyptian recipes for medications to kill pain, relieve coughs and settle the stomach. Cumin (Cuminum cyminum) is indigenous to Egypt, though the Greeks and Romans adopted it enthusiastically, and in medieval Europe it was one of the commonest spices, appearing in many recipes and remedies of the time. And it wasn't only the Scribes and Pharisees who paid their dues in cumin: any medieval English vassal who wished to avoid feudal services could include cumin as part of his 'quit rent' in lieu.

Tip

Under current UK legislation, it is illegal to uproot any wild plant without the landowner's permission, and similar laws apply elsewhere. In many parts of the world over-collection in the wild has led to the near-extinction of some popular herbs.

For example, oriental ginseng, thought to dramatically improve mental and physical well-being, is now almost extinct in the wild, as is its American counterpart. Goldenseal, once used by the Cherokee and Iroquois as a stimulating tonic and to treat many illnesses, is now said to be the most popular herbal medicine in the United States. This popularity has led to drastic over-collection in the wild, and in 1997 it was placed on the CITES II list, which forbids international trade without a licence or permit. Goldenseal has been commercially cultivated since the early twentieth century, sometimes inter-cropped with ginseng, grown for the oriental market.

The same story applies to many other herbs worldwide, so root herbs are definitely not plants to forage. Some dried roots advertised on the internet may be adulterated or misidentified, so it would be best to grow your own, or to buy dried roots from reputable, licensed organic growers, or to use commercial preparations containing root extracts.

❧ Liquorice

As children we all loved liquorice sweets.
There were the liquorice sticks and bootlaces
that stained your tongue and lips black; or
my favourite, Liquorice Allsorts, in their
pastel-coloured variety. Our parents used to
warn us that eating too many liquorice sweets
would give us 'the trots', and in fact liquorice has been used
for generations as a gentle laxative. In 1696, *The Queen's Closet
Opened* gave a liquorice, caraway and rhubarb recipe to help
'those that have not been able to go'.

As a child, I didn't connect the glossy black confectionery
with a plant, but it is made from the root of liquorice
(*Glycyrrhiza glabra*), whose genus name translates as 'sweet
root'. It is a member of the pea family, and has slightly
sticky pinnate leaves and spikes of pale violet flowers in late
summer. Liquorice comes from the eastern Mediterranean
and western Asia and was well known to the ancients.
Theophrastus called it 'sweet root' or 'Scythian root' and
said that it was good for coughs, asthma 'and in general
for troubles in the chest'. Many centuries later, people
everywhere were still taking it for coughs. The root is the
part always used, dug up when the leaves wither in late
autumn. It contains a high percentage of glycyrrhizin,
which is an astonishing fifty times sweeter than sugar.
No wonder we children enjoyed it. Liquorice
confectionery is considered safe, but
excess glycyrrhizin may cause side
effects, so don't overdo it.

There is a related wild liquorice native to northern Europe and now uncommon in Britain, but without the same medicinal virtues. True liquorice has been cultivated and valued since classical times. Liquorice is listed in the wardrobe accounts of English King Henry IV, who reigned from 1399 to 1413. A decoction of the roots was given for respiratory disorders, and as a digestive remedy. It was particularly popular as a treatment for ulcers in the mouth or the digestive tract. Clinical studies show promising results for these conditions and for dyspepsia. It is thought that liquorice extract acts in the body in a similar way to cortisone, reducing inflammation, especially in arthritis. However, taken medicinally, liquorice can raise the blood pressure and lower potassium levels, so should not be taken in high doses for periods longer than four to six weeks, and should not be used at all if you have hypertension.

Liquorice was often included in herbal recipes to mask the unpleasant taste of other ingredients, as well as bringing its own benefits. It is used in confectionery and even in stout – it adds to the flavour and colour of Guinness. In the sixteenth century, liquorice was introduced as a crop in Yorkshire, where the deep soils suited it well. Gerard grew it in his own garden and remarked that the growers in the north of England 'do manure it with great diligence'. There grew up a flourishing industry around the town of Pontefract in Yorkshire, and 'Pontefract cakes' are still well-known liquorice treats today. Nowadays imported roots are used and liquorice is no longer grown or naturalised in that area. It can be grown in temperate regions, but the tap roots can go down over a metre (3–4 feet), while the rhizomes can travel many feet sideways. The tiniest scrap left in the ground will sprout shoots, so it is not an ideal plant for a small herb garden, despite being, as Dr John Hill wrote in 1756, 'a celebrated medicine'.

Medieval French barley water
a 'sweet tea' for the sick, c.1390

I use 9 parts (by volume) of water to 1 part of pearl barley, and a 7.5cm (3in) piece of liquorice root.

Wash and strain the barley and add it to the saucepan with the fresh water and liquorice root.

Bring to the boil, then simmer together until the barley bursts (about 20 minutes).

Strain and add a dash of lemon juice.

(The writer advised feeding the cooked barley to your poultry.)

❧ Tormentil

Tormentil (*Potentilla erecta*) is well named. *Potentilla* means 'little powerful one' and 'tormentil' could come from either of two Latin words *tormentum*, meaning 'torture' or *tormina* meaning 'colic'. It is a plant that was thought to be powerful against the torture of colic, and people have treated digestive troubles with it for generations. The only inaccurate part of its name is *erecta*: it sprawls, as one writer says, 'scarce able to lift itself up'. It is common in grassland all over Europe. The rosette of basal leaves, often with five leaflets like its cousin cinquefoil (but sometimes more, hence its old name of 'septfoil'), withers before the flowers appear. The yellow flowers always have four petals and are carried on long stalks. Similar species native to other parts of the world have been used to treat the same conditions.

The red rhizome was employed in medicine, often under the alternative names of 'red-root' or 'blood-root'. The roots contain high levels of tannins, so were used to tan leather wherever tree bark was not available. Fishermen in the Scottish Islands tanned their fishing nets with red-root, too. It dyed them red, and the tannins made them last ten times longer, they said. The astringency of tormentil made it a good treatment for wounds and abrasions. The whole plant is astringent, but the roots in particular were used fresh or dried. In the seventeenth century, the juice or the powdered root was 'very effectual' either made into an ointment or spread on a plaster and applied to cuts and sores. There are records of similar use up until the twentieth century.

There is also an age-old custom in folk medicine of taking tormentil root to stop diarrhoea and dysentery. In the sixteenth century it was boiled in milk or forge water (water used to quench hot iron), then the liquid was strained and drunk. It is suggested that tormentil helped to heal the gastric condition that gave rise to diarrhoea. Tormentil contains quinoric acid, also found in *Cinchona* bark, from which quinine is made, and this could explain its other use in treating intermittent fevers which come and go like malaria. Modern herbals still advise a decoction of dried tormentil roots for mild diarrhoea, haemorrhoids, cuts and wounds. However, given that it is illegal to dig up wild plants without the landowner's permission, this is not a plant to forage. There are over-the-counter preparations containing tormentil – though be sure to follow the instructions carefully – or you might prefer other, more easily available remedies.

∾ Elecampane

Elecampane (*Inula helenium*) has been one of the most celebrated plants since earliest times. There were several legends connecting elecampane with Helen of Troy: she was holding some when 'abducted' by Paris, or she used it to heal soldiers'

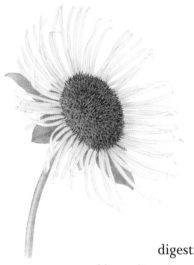

wounds, or it sprang from the earth where her tears had fallen. Elecampane's scientific name acknowledges these legends. Many ancient writers claimed that it was a remedy for snake bite, but also suggested it as a treatment for skin lesions, the digestion and most especially for coughs and lung disorders. Chinese traditional medicine used the flowers, but western traditions used only the root – though Pliny did suggest the enormous leaves, steeped in wine, as a poultice for lumbago. Roman food writer Apicius gave recipes for elecampane root in sauces and hors d'oeuvres which, he said, would help the digestion. Drinks and confectionery were flavoured with it. The big, slightly aromatic roots were candied, both as a sweetmeat and a palatable way to take one's medicine. Sugaring the pill, so to speak.

The tenth-century *Leechbook of Bald* prescribed elecampane with comfrey and honey for a dry cough. In the 1150s, Hildegard of Bingen advised a tincture of it in wine for painful lungs, and four hundred years later William Langham praised it as a treatment for 'shortness of breath, sighing and coughing'. It is known to contain around 40 per cent inulin, now an accepted medical treatment for asthma. Ever since Hippocrates, healers have been prescribing a decoction of the dried root for asthma, and it has always been a popular home remedy for bronchitis.

Elecampane also made an excellent healing wash for skin sores and to relieve the pain of neuralgia and what Galen called 'passions of the hucklebone [hip] called sciatica'. Chewing a fresh root was also supposed to fix and strengthen 'wagging teeth'. Elecampane was a great favourite with early herbalists, and appears in many Anglo-Saxon medicinal compounds. It was sometimes called 'elf-dock', from the old idea that it could treat 'elf-shot' diseases, those sudden-onset, baffling conditions that could only be explained by spiteful elves shooting you with invisible arrows.

Elecampane was brought to Britain in ancient times and has been grown in herb gardens ever since. It is tall – mine shoots up to peer over an 8-foot fence – with huge, velvety leaves and big, yellow, daisy-like flowers. It has escaped into the wild wherever it has been grown, but never spreads far from human habitation. Sometimes clumps can be found growing wild where old cottages or stables once stood. It was used to medicate horses in Britain and the US up until the twentieth century, which accounts for another vernacular name: 'horseheal'.

One prominent modern herbalist recommends making a cold infusion of elecampane root by steeping one teaspoonful of shredded root in a cup of cold water overnight, then straining it. He suggests taking this, hot, three times a day for respiratory conditions, though unless you are prepared to sacrifice a plant from your garden, you will have to buy ready-dried root.

∾ Juniper

We always refer to
juniper fruits as berries.
Common juniper (*Juniperus
communis*) is a dioecious conifer, so
the 'berries' are in fact female cones,
while the male flowers are little tufts of yellow stamens on
a separate plant. The berries are green in their first year,
only ripening in their second or even third year, so there are
always ripe and unripe berries on the same branch. Common
juniper grows in temperate and arctic areas around the
northern hemisphere, and people everywhere have always
found it useful. It used to be widespread in Britain – in the
seventeenth century it was 'plentiful' – but it is now local and
declining. There are several subspecies and many cultivars, as
well as related species around the world.

Like many conifers, juniper is aromatic and its timber
was made into moth-proof chests and boxes. The smoke
from burning juniper wood was considered both special and
beneficial, and at least three ancient European physicians
wrote recipes for juniper incense cakes. People from the
Arapaho to traditional healers in Tibet, and even French
nurses in the Second World War, burned it to fumigate and
disinfect sickrooms and to treat patients.

The part most often used in medicine, however, was the
berries. They contain an oil which is stimulant, carminative,
antiseptic and strongly diuretic, so helpful in treating
cystitis, dropsy and digestive disorders. It was thought to be
good for coughs and colds and, made into a poultice, was

used to help heal wounds and ulcers on the skin. Culpeper couldn't praise it highly enough, saying it 'can scarcely be equalled for its virtues'. However, it stimulates the nephrons strongly, so people with kidney disease should not take it.

Juniper is enjoyed as a culinary ingredient, of course, especially with rich meats and game. But, historically, it was best known as an abortifacient. There is a very long oral tradition of this application, and one brutally straightforward country name for it was 'bastard-killer'. In 1694, physician John Pechey wrote that it was 'too well known and too much used by wenches'. It was not only poor women who had recourse to juniper. A Tudor ballad relates the sad tale of one of Mary Queen of Scots' ladies who tried to procure an abortion with juniper. The attempt failed and she was beheaded. Juniper's reputation continued for centuries and illicit preparations were available under the counter at some pharmacies until well into the twentieth century. Needless to say, juniper is not safe to take during pregnancy, and certainly not to encourage abortion.

Juniper oil should only be taken under expert supervision, but there are many who will add a few berries to food or make them into drinks. Theophrastus said they tasted 'remarkably fragrant' and they were sometimes chewed to freshen the breath. The ancient Egyptians used an infusion of berries for indigestion and wind, though, according to Gerard, too much would give you 'gripings and gnawings in the stomach'. It will also colour your urine violet, say some, or make it smell of violets, say others. I have yet to determine which is accurate.

Juniper soak for arthritic hands

Put one teaspoonful of lightly crushed berries into a mug and pour on boiling water.

Cover and infuse for 10 minutes.

Then pour into a bowl of hot (but not scalding) water and soak the painful hands for 20 minutes.

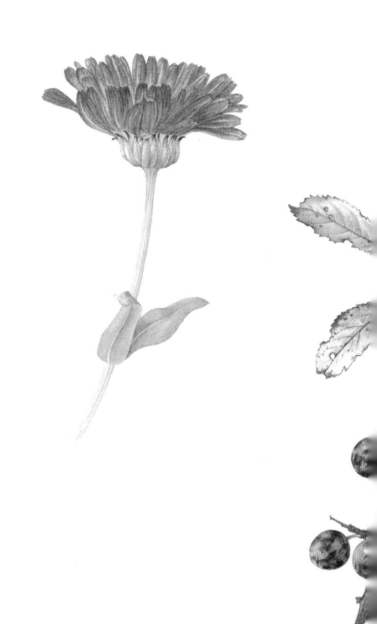

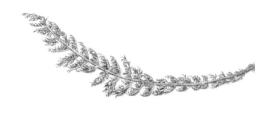

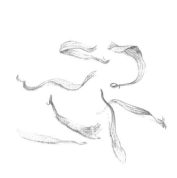

Winter

The struggling winter howling by

JOHN CLARE (1793–1864),
The Shepherd's Calendar

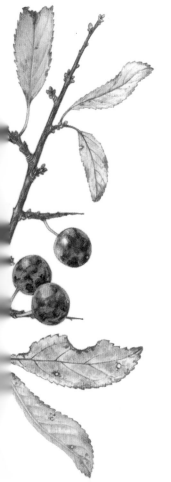

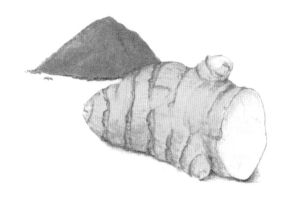

As the winter weather closes in, we more often fall prey to ailments and discomforts, such as chilblains, colds and flu, or rheumatic aches and pains. And in winter there are fewer fresh plant remedies to be found. Even evergreens such as rosemary are more potent if picked just before flowering. So the wise would have collected herbs in season and dried or preserved them for winter. Some herbs are included here because, while they flower in the summer, they are so useful in dried or preserved form in winter. Down the centuries, every household would have had a medicine cupboard full of these remedies and first aid treatments. And when using them in the cold, dark days of winter, it is comforting to remember harvesting them in the summer sunshine.

∾ Rosemary

Being evergreen, rosemary (*Rosmarinus officinalis*) symbolised everlasting life. It became associated with remembrance – poor, deranged Ophelia says: 'there's rosemary, that's for remembrance' – and it was used in memorial offerings at funerals, a tradition that continues to this day: the late Queen Elizabeth II's coffin bore a wreath which included rosemary. On the other hand, it was also thought to ensure the long happiness of newly married couples. Tudor royal brides carried rosemary, and it played a part in marriage customs until Victorian times. As Robert Herrick observed in his 1648 poem 'The Rosemarie Branch':

> Grow for two ends, it matters not at all,
> Be't for my Bridall, or my Buriall.

As well as flavouring food – and its mild antibiotic properties may have protected diners from suspect meats, as well as masking their flavour – rosemary has always been used medicinally. At the Royal Maundy ceremony, when money is distributed to elderly commoners, the British sovereign still today carries a nosegay that includes rosemary. The posy symbolically protects against infection, a reminder of the days when Maundy recipients might well have been carrying infectious diseases. Rosemary was thought a powerful

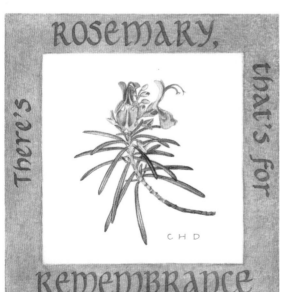

protection against the plague, and in his pamphlet *The Wonderfull Yeare* (1603, a plague year) Thomas Dekker sourly remarked that 'rosemary, which had wont to be sold for twelve pence an armful, went now at six shillings a handful'. Nothing changes!

Rosemary grows wild in dry, stony ground around the Mediterranean. Its name comes from Latin words meaning 'dew of the sea', as it flourished on cliffs. In the sixteenth century, it was said to be so plentiful in Languedoc, southern France, that the local people used nothing but rosemary for their firewood. It must have smelled lovely. Rosemary has always been grown in herb gardens, and it probably arrived in Britain with the Romans. Fifteenth-century advice was that in England it should be grown in pots that could be brought under cover in winter, but it survives happily enough outside all year in my garden in the south of England. As far as I know, it has not yet escaped into the wild in these latitudes.

Gerard writes that 'the Arabians and other Physicians succeeding, do write, that rosemary comforts the brain, the memory, the inward senses, and restores speech unto them that are possessed with the dumb palsy'. Rosemary was often included in preparations to counter melancholy, too. Perhaps its symbolic connection with remembrance suggested it as a treatment for poor memory, but it does contain the flavonoid diosmin, known to strengthen blood vessels and aid circulation; so it may help by improving blood flow to the head and stimulating the nervous system.

Rosemary's action as a circulatory stimulant might help with physical aches and pains, too. I have massaged cold, aching joints and muscles with rosemary-infused oil, and have found my circulation improved by taking an infusion, one teaspoonful of chopped herb to a cup of boiling water. But don't drink it just before bedtime or it may keep you awake. Also, highly concentrated extracts may interact with some medications, so check with your doctor before taking them.

Our grandmothers used rosemary as a hair tonic, especially for dark hair. A final rinse with a strong infusion of rosemary will give the hair a lovely shine. One modern herbalist recommends massaging a dry scalp with rosemary-infused oil half an hour before shampooing. Today, many commercial shampoos contain rosemary, partly for its conditioning qualities and partly for its lovely fresh smell.

✺ Wintergreen

Those of us who are getting on in years are likely to suffer with stiff, aching joints due to rheumatism or arthritis, especially in winter. The same was true of our forebears, and a great many remedies were suggested in folk traditions and written in herbals. One of the most popular in recent centuries was Oil of Wintergreen. Massaged into the affected limb, it would ease the pain, and even its penetrating smell suggested that it must be doing you good. Extracts are still used today to perfume products such as toothpaste and shampoo.

There are many closely related species of wintergreen growing over a huge geographical range, but the medicinal plant is *Gaultheria procumbens*, an American native shrub. Often growing in damp, acid woodland, it is low-growing, spreading and evergreen, with white bell-like flowers in the summer and red berries that last all winter. The leaves used

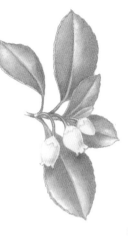

to be listed in the official US Pharmacopoeia, but by the 1930s only the oil extracted from them remained on the list. Frosted, purple leaves were said to yield the most oil.

Wintergreen is native to the eastern parts of North America, and the Algonquin and Iroquois people, among others, took it as an anti-rheumatic and a cold remedy. Early settlers learned its value from them and it soon became familiar to herbalists in Europe. However, the name caused considerable confusion, as there is a group of distantly related European native plants, also called wintergreens, in the *Pyrola* genus.

Nicholas Culpeper describes wintergreen (*Gaultheria*) as a treatment for conditions affecting several internal organs and says it 'taketh away any inflammation rising upon pains of the heart'. This makes sense, as the essential oil contained in the leaves is 99 per cent methyl salicylate, very similar to aspirin and with the same pain-relieving and anti-inflammatory properties. And today aspirin is prescribed to thin the blood and reduce inflammation in cardiovascular conditions.

Wintergreen should not be used internally, as it can be toxic in excess. In addition, the natural oil applied externally can cause skin problems, so it is perhaps advisable to treat yourself with the synthetic wintergreen oil available over the counter and just enjoy wintergreen itself as an attractive garden plant.

❧ Marigold

Since at least the Middle Ages, an
essential for every household's winter
store cupboard was dried marigold petals.
This was the common or pot marigold (Calendula officinalis),
not the French, African or Mexican marigolds, which
are Tagetes species, nor the native marsh marigold (Caltha
palustris), whose big, yellow, buttercup flowers stud marshes
and stream-sides in the spring. I mean the plant with soft,
light-green leaves and big, vibrant-orange, daisy-like flowers.

The name 'marigold' is supposed to derive from 'Mary's
Gold', to distinguish the medicinally valuable Calendula from
the similar-looking cornfield weed Glebionis segetum, which
was historically called simply 'gold'. Just to confuse matters,
this cornfield weed is now called 'corn marigold', illustrating
once again the treachery of common names. Gerard suggests
that the scientific name Calendula comes from the fact that
marigolds flower on the calends (first day) of almost every
month: 'It flowers from April or May even until winter, and
in winter also, if it be warm.'

The Romans used marigold petals as a cheap substitute for
saffron, and for centuries cooks used them to add colour to
butter, cheese and cakes. The petals are rich in carotenoids,
which impart a yellow colour. If your hair colour was not to
your liking, you could make it more golden with a rinse of
marigold petal infusion.

It is uncertain exactly where marigolds originated, but
they were cultivated in gardens everywhere from India to
Britain for many centuries, often escaping into the wild

and looking startlingly exotic among the wayside weeds. Their brilliant orange flowers lift the spirits, and people thought that just looking at them 'drove evil humours out of the head', and even strengthened the eyesight. The French herbalist known as Floridus Macer wrote in the eleventh century: 'The golden flower is good to be seen, it makes the sight bright and clean.' The distilled juice was recommended as eye drops for inflammation, but certainly we know today never to put anything in the eye without first taking medical advice.

I always thought that the name 'pot marigold' arose from the practice of growing it in pots, but in fact it is because it was often used in the cooking pot. In sixteenth-century 'Dutchland' (the Netherlands and Germany), merchants sold huge quantities of dried marigold petals in winter, both for medicinal preparations and to add colour and flavour to food. No broths were considered well made without them.

Marigolds close their flowers at night. In *A Winter's Tale*, Shakespeare refers to: 'The marigold that goes to bed wi' th' sun, and with him rises, weeping' – presumably weeping with dew. Like sunflowers, they turn their faces to follow the sun. Because of their apparent devotion to the sun, marigolds became a symbol of constancy in love, and the petals were even thought to be an aphrodisiac. I often think of this when adding their colourful petals to a salad.

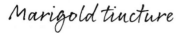

Marigold tincture

15g (½ oz) fresh petals (or half this quantity of dried petals)

200ml (7fl oz) alcohol, such as vodka or brandy

6 tablespoons distilled water

Chop or bruise the petals and put into a large jar.

Mix the alcohol and water together and add to the jar. Cover and label with the date.

Leave in a dark place for two weeks, shaking well every day. Don't be tempted to leave it longer: it won't get any stronger and the herb will start to break down.

Strain through a sieve (strainer) lined with muslin (cheesecloth). Squeeze the cloth to extract every drop of goodness.

Pour into a sterilised dark glass bottle and label with the dose required. In a clean bottle, a tincture should last almost indefinitely.

I use one teaspoonful, diluted in a glass of water, as a gargle for sore throats, or as a wash or compress for cuts, grazes and stings. It should not be used internally during pregnancy or lactation, and not at all by people who are allergic to plants in the Asteraceae (daisy) family.

More practically, infusions of petals and leaves were used internally to treat jaundice, sore throats, fevers and more serious illnesses, too. In 1699, while away from home, Sir John Clerk received a letter from his wife telling him that their son had contracted smallpox and that she was giving him marigold posset to drink. How interesting that even a wealthy family would use simple remedies, as well as the complicated, multi-ingredient, sometimes brutal (and no doubt expensive) treatments prescribed by the physicians of the day.

Marigold has always been applied externally to treat wounds and many different skin conditions. Antiseptic and anti-fungal, it was highly thought of by American surgeons, who used it to treat wounds during the Civil War. I make an antiseptic tincture with the petals to treat cuts and grazes.

☙ Arnica

Throughout history, people have sought first aid for swellings and contusions – or, as Gerard put it, 'any bruise, black or blue spots gotten by falls, or women's wilfulness in stumbling upon their hasty husband's fists, or such like'. He went on to prescribe a remedy popular at the time: a poultice made from the fresh roots of Solomon's seal. It would, he said, take away the bruising in one night, or two at the most.

Nowadays, the treatment we reach for is often based on arnica. My own doctor surprised me recently when, following an accident, he checked me for broken bones and then recommended arnica cream for the extensive bruising. A physiotherapist friend confirmed that massaging bruises prevents calcification deep within the tissue, and the arnica was an added bonus.

Arnica (*Arnica montana*) is indigenous to the mountains of central Europe, but is now grown everywhere the climate allows, as an attractive garden plant. Its sunny yellow flowers bloom in summer, but are useful year round in preserved form. Since at least the fifteenth century, people in Europe and Russia used the root and the flowers medicinally, making a tincture into an ointment or cream for external application. It was taken internally, too, to reduce fevers and inflammation. However, internal use is no longer recommended, as its irritation to the stomach can prove dangerous or even fatal. Homeopathic doses, where the concentration is very low, are safe to take internally for bruising; but there is no medical evidence that they have much effect. There is some evidence that arnica applied externally is safe and effective, supporting years of folk tradition, though it should not be used on broken skin or during pregnancy or lactation, or by people with an allergy to the daisy family.

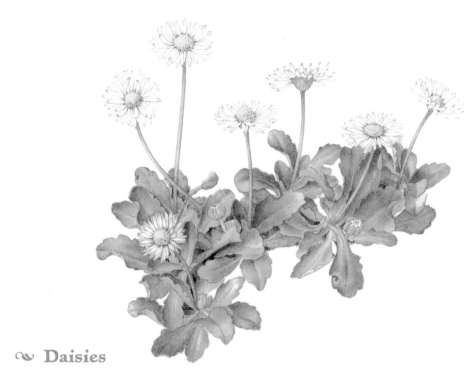

∾ Daisies

In western Europe, we had our own remedy for bruising
in the common daisy (*Bellis perennis*). It is very common
indeed – the Royal Horticultural Society describes it as
'ubiquitous' – so it is rarely grown in gardens, at least not
intentionally. The scientific name comes from the Latin
bellus, meaning 'pretty'; and to me, any lawn should be
spangled with what poet Robert Burns called a 'bonny gem'.
Children love making daisy chains and playing 'he loves me,
he loves me not …' with daisy petals. It was a favourite of
Geoffrey Chaucer, who pointed out that its name comes from
'Day's Eye', as it closes up at night. There was an old saying
that spring had arrived when you could put your foot on
seven daisies. Sterner folk said twelve; the more optimistic
said three. Although the flowers are a welcome sign of spring,
the leaves provided a standby remedy throughout the year.

Daisy leaves and roots have been made into ointments for wounds and bruises since Chaucer's day, and probably long before that – an old name for it was 'bruisewort'. Physicians also prescribed a poultice of pounded leaves for bruises. The leaves contain a juice so acrid that cattle and even insects refuse to eat them – how often do you see caterpillar holes in a daisy leaf? – but this astringency was thought to be helpful in healing wounds. Gerard claimed that 'the juice of the leaves and roots sniffed up into the nostrils, purges the head mightily, and helps the megrim [migraine]'. Before snorting daisy juice for a migraine, I think I would try kinder remedies, such as feverfew. But, if I had run out of arnica cream, I might apply a poultice of daisy leaves to a bruise.

Witch hazel

It is often said that witch hazel's name has less to do with witches and more to do with the use of its flexible twigs for switches or whips. That said, several of its European vernacular names also hint at magic. The trees that brighten our winter gardens with their delightful, often fragrant, spidery yellow flowers are mainly varieties developed from the Chinese *Hamamelis mollis*, but the species used medicinally is *Hamamelis virginiana*, a small, native woodland or forest-edge tree of the eastern United States. Its flowers are less showy than the garden varieties, and appear in the autumn, just as the leaves are turning gold.

The Iroquois, Mohegan and other tribes traditionally made a decoction of the twigs or bark, and used it internally and externally to treat inflammations, stop bleeding, and relieve coughs and colds. The early colonists soon adopted the remedy and found a compress of witch hazel to be an excellent treatment for bruises, bleeding and varicose veins. Very diluted, it made a good eyewash for conjunctivitis. Made into an ointment or suppositories, it was an effective treatment for piles. Being so full of tannins, it has an astringent effect useful in all such conditions.

In the mid-nineteenth century, a commercially produced extract of witch hazel was marketed as Pond's Extract or Witch Hazel Water. It soon became very popular on both sides of the Atlantic, and our grandmothers always had a bottle in the cupboard for emergencies. Similar products are still available today, though they should only be used externally.

∽ Puffballs, cobwebs and sphagnum moss

Our ancestors used all sorts of things as first aid for cuts and wounds. The main objective was to stop the bleeding, of course, preferably while preventing infection. Many summer herbs, when applied fresh, fulfilled both roles very well, but in the winter people turned to dried medicine-chest standbys, including puffballs.

Puffballs (*Lycoperdon* spp and *Calvatia* spp) are a group of fungi which, when mature, expel their spores through a hole in the top, rather than through gills or pores under a cap. Most are pear- or club-shaped, and the best known of all is the giant puffball (*Clavatia gigantia*), a big white ball which can be 30cm (12in) or more in diameter. Puffballs grow in woods or sometimes on heaths in temperate latitudes all around the northern hemisphere. There are records of the Lakota and Blackfoot in North America using them as styptic remedies which would prevent infection, and puffballs are also mentioned as an effective wound treatment in some of the old European herbals.

In eighteenth- and nineteenth-century England, butchers, carpenters and blacksmiths always kept some at the ready to treat the cuts inevitable in their trades. Some people collected young puffballs and dried slices ready for emergencies, while others used mature fungi, tearing off a strip to apply like a plaster (band-aid), with the spore side next to the wound. Still others dried the whole fungus and puffed the spores into the wound when needed. There is some medical evidence confirming their efficacy.

Many puffballs are good to eat when young and firm, but take care not to confuse them with the superficially similar-looking earth balls (*Scleroderma* spp), which are poisonous. Until quite recently, the sensible French trained their pharmacists in fungus recognition, and there were charts in every pharmacy illustrating which of your foraged fungi were dangerous and which would make a delicious meal.

Another wound treatment with a very long folk tradition is the spider's web. It has a reputation for being antiseptic and anti-fungal – so long as it is clean, and not full of dust, like most of the cobwebs in my house. Outdoor webs would probably be best. Salt, too, is well known as a wound-healer, as sailors and surfers will confirm, and many people find that a salty water mouthwash helps to heal mouth ulcers.

Although sphagnum moss is known to have been applied as a wound dressing since early times, none of the ancient or medieval herbal writers mention it. They do occasionally write about 'moss', but from their descriptions I have an uneasy feeling that they are actually talking about lichen. If they do mean moss, it certainly isn't sphagnum. *Sphagnum* mosses grow in wet, acid, boggy places around the world, in temperate and even tundra regions. Another name for the whole group is 'bog-mosses'. Their structure allows them to hold huge amounts of water.

When dried, sphagnum is lightweight and super-absorbent. This, combined with its proven antiseptic properties, made it a very valuable field-wound dressing. There are records of its use on battlefields from at least the eleventh century (Battle of Clontarf, Ireland, 1014). In the First World War, large-scale collection by the public began in 1914, and both sides in the conflict made use of sphagnum dressings. Sadly, sphagnum is declining, partly due to habitat loss, but also through over-collection for the horticulture trade. Fresh sphagnum is sold to line hanging baskets, and decayed sphagnum is the main constituent of peat, overused in gardening everywhere.

～ Aloe

There are several hundred *Aloe* species, ranging from large trees to small succulent rosettes. They all originate in Africa, the Middle East and the Mediterranean. I have visited a tall aloe tree revered as a sacred site in a village in Madagascar, while many smaller species are grown as attractive houseplants in cooler regions. Cape aloe (*Aloe ferox*) and the well-known *Aloe vera* are the two most often used medicinally.

The name 'aloe' comes from a Hebrew word meaning 'bitter', and two medicines are produced: 'drug aloe', a very bitter juice extracted from the leaf bases, and 'aloe gel', which exudes from the broken leaves. The juice has always been given as a powerful emetic and laxative, far too drastic for modern home use. It was among the remedies recommended to Alfred the Great by the Patriarch of Jerusalem in the ninth century. Even the most exalted were plainly made of stronger stuff in those days. As a child, I used to bite my fingernails, until my mother painted them with 'bitter aloe'. It proved a very effective deterrent. Aloe gel is an excellent treatment for skin conditions and small injuries, especially burns and

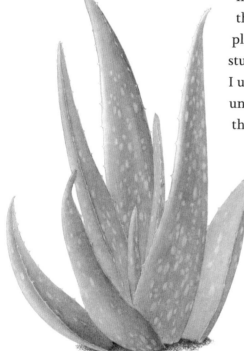

scalds. Medical research now confirms this, though down the ages wise people everywhere have kept an aloe in the home for use in emergencies. It isn't known as the 'first aid plant' for nothing. Commercially produced aloe gel is now available, but the extraction process may use harsh chemicals, and the gel may be adulterated with other ingredients. I simply break a leaf in half and apply the gel directly onto the affected area. *Aloe vera* is very easy to grow and propagate, so first aid can always be at hand.

∾ Senna and cascara

Another essential standby in the medicine cabinet would be a treatment for constipation, and the most popular was senna. Senna belongs to a large genus of leguminous plants originating in Africa, Egypt, Arabia and India. Until recently, it was classified as a member of the *Cassia* genus, whose range also includes Asia and the Americas. There is some evidence that people everywhere used their own indigenous species in much the same way, as a laxative. European colonists in Australia planted attractive, fragrant cassia bushes to screen the outside earth closet, or 'dunny', and the plant is affectionately known by some as 'dunny-bush'. Even today, you can often see isolated cassia bushes standing apart from rural homesteads, marking where the dunny once stood.

The best-known species of senna is Alexandrian senna (*Senna alexandrina*). It was written about by Arab physicians such as Serapion the Elder in the tenth century, though it had no doubt been valued in folk medicine for a long time before that. It is still grown commercially, particularly in India. Theophrastus gives a detailed description of the harvesting of cassia bark in the Arabian Peninsula, but it is senna leaves – and more especially the pods – that are generally used today.

Early physicians recognised senna's purgative properties, but also its 'nauseous taste' and tendency to cause griping and even vomiting. So they recommended adding aromatic ingredients to the mixture, both to disguise the taste and to ease the discomfort of the remedial process. For example, a 1639 book, The Charitable Physician, suggested a senna infusion that also included cinnamon, liquorice, aniseed and ginger among other things.

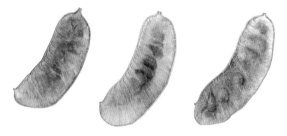

Senna is an ingredient of many over-the-counter remedies, and dried pods can be bought if you prefer to make your own infusion. Both are used in the short term to relieve constipation. There was – and unfortunately still is – a widespread belief that frequent purging is good for the system, or aids weight loss. Neither is true, and long-term use of laxatives can cause serious harm.

The store-cupboard laxative of choice in North America was often cascara sagrada, or Californian buckthorn (Frangula *purshiana*). The Costanoan, Mahuna and Pomo peoples, among others, gave the berries or dried bark as a laxative infusion. Older bark was thought to be gentler and less likely to cause vomiting, though the taste was still unpleasantly bitter.

Californian buckthorn is a relative of the European purging buckthorn (*Rhamnus cathartica*) – also a powerful purgative, as both its scientific and common names indicate. Buckthorn seeds found in excavations of medieval monastery waste pits suggest that the monks were using the berries to relieve constipation. By the sixteenth century, the berries were considered too drastic a treatment for humans, but suitable for horses. Now they are no longer even given to horses.

❧ Sloes, blackthorn

After a long, dark winter, the first white blossoms in the hedgerows are a welcome sign that spring is on its way. Many people assume that all early blossom is blackthorn (*Prunus spinosa*), but in fact its close relative the cherry plum (*Prunus cerasifera*) usually flowers first, sometimes as early as January. Blackthorn follows a little later. Its flowers, clustered along the twigs, smell of almonds and have a sharp, slightly bitter taste. According to Mrs Grieve, an infusion of flowers was occasionally given to children as a gentle purgative. This is slightly alarming to hear, as the flowers and young leaves contain a cyanide compound, which accounts for the smell and taste.

Blackthorn is one of several European wild plums and is thought to be one of the parents of *Prunus domestica*, the origin of all our cultivated plums. The various species do hybridise freely, so exact identification can be tricky, but our ancestors used all the wild plums in much the same way. Gerard wrote that a larger-fruited variety grew near Damascus, 'a town in Syria', and was known as the 'damascene plum' or 'damson'.

Blackthorn attracted a good deal of folklore – bringing the blossom indoors invited a death, or that witches favoured blackthorn walking sticks, for instance – but it was not much valued in healing, apart from the fruits, or 'sloes'. Two hundred years ago, in *Rural Rides*, William Cobbett wrote of eating raw sloes as a boy 'until my tongue clove to the roof of my mouth and my lips were pretty near glued together', so astringent was the juice. Because of this astringency, people used sloes to treat bleeding and diarrhoea. Sloes were dried for use in winter, as advised in the country rhyme:

At the end of October go gather up sloes,
Have thou in readiness plenty of those,
And keep them in bedstraw or still on the bough
to stay both the flux of thyself and thy cow.

Flux or lask (diarrhoea) and the bloody flux (dysentery) were
very common in less hygienic times, and an effective, freely
available remedy would have been very welcome.

Sloes are still valued nowadays, though not for medicine.
Country people have always collected the small, sour, blue–
black berries to make a useful dye and an excellent
marking-ink, as well as cooking them in pies,
jams and jellies. And, of course, to make sloe
wine and sloe gin. It was said that, if you
could keep your hands off sloe wine for a
year or two, it would come to resemble
a fine port in taste and colour. I never
managed to keep it long enough, and the
sloe gin never lasted beyond Christmas.

◌ Slippery elm

Our grandmothers used to talk of 'slippery elm food' as
excellent nourishment for young children and invalids. It
was sold as a powder and mixed with water to make a kind of
gruel or porridge, perhaps with cinnamon or sugar added to
improve the taste. It comes from the 'bast' or inner bark of
the North American elm tree Ulmus rubra, also known as 'red
elm' and 'moose elm'. It is a tall tree with reddish leaves in

the spring and is native to the central and southern United States. The bast (pale and slimy, hence the vernacular name) is collected in the spring, then dried and powdered. When mixed with water, it expands in a similar way to flax seed, and its mucilage could soothe and relieve a variety of ills.

It could be made into a thick, soothing tea for internal use. With less water it was considered to be an excellent poultice for external use with or without other herbs. And it was indeed very nutritious. The Cherokee and Iroquois, among others, took it to soothe sore throats and calm the digestive tract, while some, such as the Micmac, also made poultices for sores and wounds. Many Native American peoples appear to have esteemed it highly.

Slippery elm is still sold today for the treatment of sore throats. Some find it soothes and lubricates the whole digestive system, too, relieving the discomfort of ulcers and inflammation. It was even used as an enema in cases of constipation. But, historically, it was sometimes also employed by desperate women who found themselves 'in trouble'. As such, it is definitely not a herb to be used when pregnant.

The popularity of slippery elm has led to conservation issues, as collection of the inner bark often kills the tree. Some slippery elm powder includes the outer bark, which is a much less effective medication. Like so many elms, *Ulmus rubra* has succumbed to Dutch elm disease. The Royal Horticultural Society of London reports that the disease has destroyed almost all European and American native elm trees since the mid-1960s, and despite valiant efforts by arboriculturists, no truly disease-resistant hybrids have yet been found.

∾ Cloves

We often underestimate the amount of international
trade there was even in early times. Merchants brought
silks, spices – and ideas – from far-off places along well-
established trading routes for thousands of years. In fourth
century BCE Athens, Theophrastus described in detail
the harvesting and preparation of cinnamon from Arabia
and other spices from India. The Romans were familiar
with pepper, cinnamon, ginger, cloves and many other
exotic commodities. The Roman Empire played a part
in distributing these goods, of course, and by the eighth
century CE foreign-grown spices were known all over
northern Europe, and were mentioned in descriptions
of dishes and medicines. Weary fighters returning from
the Crusades may have brought exotic culinary souvenirs
home with them, too. By the thirteenth century,
physicians such as Arnau de Villanova were recommending
sauces made with these warming spices for winter health
and well-being. And don't nutmeg, cinnamon, ginger and
cloves still smell of Christmas and cosy winter comforts to
us today?

At first only the wealthy could afford such luxury goods.
Spices were one of the prizes that spurred exploration,
started wars and made Venetian and Dutch traders very
wealthy. The spice trade was also one of the drivers that
led to colonisation. As easier sea routes opened up, and
plantations were established closer to home – often by

stealing seeds or cuttings from under the noses of the original producers – prices began to drop and spices became more available to everyone.

Cloves are the dried, unopened flower buds of a tropical tree, *Syzygium aromaticum*, which originally grew only in the Moluccas. These islands, now known as Maluku, are part of Indonesia, but were known for centuries – rather excitingly – as the Spice Islands. The name 'clove' comes from the Latin *clavus*, meaning 'nail'. By the seventeenth century, most households would have kept some cloves to use in cooking and as medicine, or even to make a pomander for sweetening the air. When I was a child in the 1950s, we made pomanders at Christmas. We studded oranges with cloves and rolled them in spices such as cinnamon and nutmeg, with powdered orris root to fix the perfume. They remained fragrant all year.

Cloves have an analgesic and anti-inflammatory effect well known in ancient India and China. For generations, people in Europe have applied the strongly antiseptic oil of cloves particularly to relieve toothache and inflamed gums. If the oil was not available, a clove gently chewed, or even simply held in the mouth, would have the same effect. Clove oil contains the compound eugenol, which is responsible for its aromatic and beneficial effects; but ingested in large amounts, it can damage the liver.

Eighteenth-century ladies used a clove, charred in a candle flame, as an eyebrow pencil. When I tried this, the clove caught fire and I had to quickly blow it out. But it did make a lovely soft brown once it had cooled.

❧ Ginger

One stormy January day, when about to embark on a ferry crossing to France, one of my companions offered me some crystallised ginger, saying it would stop me being seasick. She had spent many years at sea with her sailor husband, and always had ginger to hand for when nausea threatened. I didn't know it at the time, but she was following an age-old custom, as ginger (Zingiber officinale) has a very long-standing reputation for settling nausea and vomiting. Recent scientific trials appear to confirm its efficacy against motion sickness, and suggest it may even help with nausea and vomiting due to pregnancy or chemotherapy, though more research is needed. I can, however, report that I survived the ferry crossing without incident.

Many early writers also recommended ginger as a carminative treatment for colic and flatulence. Dioscorides said it was 'stomach-warming' and would 'soften the intestines gently'. It was sometimes added to laxative preparations to ameliorate the harsh effects of other ingredients.

Originating in maritime parts of tropical South-East Asia, ginger was taken into cultivation and spread in ancient times to China, India and the Pacific islands. It was important in medicine and cuisine in both the Ayurvedic and Chinese traditions. Confucius (551–478 BCE) was said to have eaten it with every meal, and a friend who worked in a British centre for Vietnamese refugees in the 1970s told me that the grocery lists always included large quantities of ginger. In 406 CE the Buddhist monk Faxian reported that potted ginger plants were carried on Chinese ships to prevent scurvy. Ginger root does contain some vitamin C, and traditional Chinese medicine prescribed an infusion of ginger leaves for nausea – so perhaps it served as a seasickness remedy, too.

Arab traders brought ginger to Europe and the Romans introduced it all over their empire. It was very highly valued everywhere: Pliny wrote that 'both ginger and pepper grow wild in their own countries, yet they are purchased by weight as if they were gold or silver'. It remained expensive for centuries: in fourteenth-century England a pound of ginger cost the same as a sheep. European settlers brought ginger to the Americas, where it was cultivated and then exported back to Europe. A North American native plant called wild ginger (*Asarum canadense*) is in fact a distant relative of root ginger and it was used medicinally in similar ways.

As a child, I rarely saw ginger as a fresh root (technically a rhizome, an underground stem); much more often it appeared as a powder used in baking, as a wizened little dried thing used in pickling, as delicious crystallised lumps or as luscious 'stem ginger' in jars of syrup. But how we loved it! Ginger biscuits, dark sticky ginger cake and those green bottles of ginger wine, perfect for a cold winter's evening, were perennial favourites.

Ginger is a circulatory stimulant, 'gingering up' the system. Whether taken as a tea, used in hand and foot baths or made into an infused oil rub, it will warm up cold, aching extremities. I make a massage oil (below) with ginger and other warming ingredients.

'Winter Warmer' massage oil

Into a clean glass jam jar slice about 4–5cm (1½–2in) of ginger root (or 2 teaspoons of dried ginger). Add 3–4 tablespoons of cayenne pepper, 2 tablespoons of mustard powder and a teaspoon or two of ground black pepper.

Pour in about 300ml (½ pint) of sunflower or rapeseed oil and put on the lid.

Warm gently in a bain-marie (water bath) for 2 hours or so.

Strain through a sieve (strainer) lined with muslin (cheesecloth), and pour into a clean bottle. Don't forget to label it.

I use the beautiful, orange-coloured oil to massage stiff, cold hands and feet, but have a care as, while the capsaicin in the cayenne acts to relieve arthritic pain, it can irritate broken skin. And remember not to rub your eyes after applying it!

∾ Mallows

Like many children before me, I used to munch the
immature fruits (known as 'cheeses') of common mallow
(*Malva sylvestris*) on my way home from school. They
reminded me of green, curled-up caterpillars, but I liked
the slightly nutty taste. I recently read that they have a
mild laxative effect, though I can't say I noticed that at the

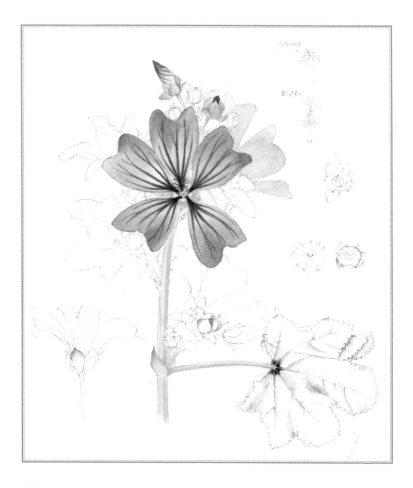

time. Common mallow belongs to a genus of plants related to hollyhocks, hibiscus, okra and cotton. I always liked the mauve, trumpet-shaped flowers, streaked with darker lines, and the paler flowers of its close relative musk mallow, with its finely divided leaves. Both grow on roadsides and well-drained waste ground. On seaside holidays I sometimes saw the stately tree mallow, too. Mallow species are native to Eurasia and North Africa, but have now been introduced worldwide. They all contain a great deal of mucilage, and so people employed them both internally and externally for wounds, soreness and inflammation, as well as for food. Archaeological evidence from the Middle East and the Balkans suggests that we have been using mallows for thousands of years, and there are records of its continuing folk use everywhere it grows.

A friend's grandmother used to insist that any mallow leaf, laid on the skin and held there with a handkerchief, would draw out thorns and splinters. Pliny said the same thing 2,000 years ago. When I related this connection to a botanist friend, he told me that on a field trip to Madagascar a local botanist colleague got a long, thin thorn embedded in his hand and went off to look for a particular plant to treat it. He came back with a leaf that my friend said looked very like either a mallow or a hibiscus leaf, broke the central vein and squeezed the sap onto his hand. The following morning he showed my friend that the thorn was protruding just enough to grasp and pull it out.

The healing properties of mallows have been recorded in an unbroken tradition since classical antiquity. Horace and Virgil both mention them, as do Dioscorides and several early Arab physicians. Bald's tenth-century *Leechbook* prescribes mallow leaf to heal blood-letting incisions that have become infected. Culpeper wrote in 1649 that mallow roots were 'full of a slimy juice which being laid in water will thicken it as if it were jelly'. This mucilage, which also has antibacterial properties, was made into poultices that healed wounds, drew boils and soothed inflamed skin very effectively. In the nineteenth century, teething babies were still given mallow stalks or roots to chew on. A modern French herbal advises mallow-leaf infusions as a gargle for a sore throat, by the spoonful for a cough, and by the cupful for constipation.

The dried leaves were sometimes boiled in water to make a wound treatment. William Cobbett remarked in *Rural Rides*: 'its operation in all cases is so quick that it is hardly to be believed'; he went on to describe several cases he had witnessed personally. He urged everyone to collect and dry plenty of mallow leaves for use in winter, adding, 'now a person must be almost criminally careless not to make provision of this herb'. Although it flowers all summer, it is a staple of the winter medicine cabinet.

As well as healing the outside, mallow remedies were taken to treat inner ailments, too. Their soothing, demulcent effect helped with inflammations of the digestive system and chest complaints. They were made into a variety of preparations to treat coughs and sore throats. Dried mallow flowers were one ingredient of the old French cough remedy *tisane de quatre fleurs*, infused together with flowers of sweet violet, mullein (*Verbascum*) and poppy petals. Nicholas Culpeper wrote: 'Pliny says, that whosoever shall take a spoonful of any of the mallows, shall that day be free from all diseases that may come unto him.'

Early authors did not discriminate between the different mallows, but gradually marsh mallow (Althaea officinalis), became the species preferred for medicinal use. It has even more mucilage than its relatives, so was more often listed as the official herb in later herbals, as its specific name suggests. However, marsh mallow is uncommon in Britain, so most people continued to use common mallow in home medicine, as is borne out in surviving records of the oral tradition. Scientific studies confirm that all the mallows are safe to consume, and in southern Europe common mallow is often added to soups and stews. In the late eighteenth century, French confectioners made the first marshmallow sweets – health lozenges combining marsh mallow root jelly, sugar and egg whites. Sadly, the marshmallows on sale today are made with gelatine and contain no mallow at all.

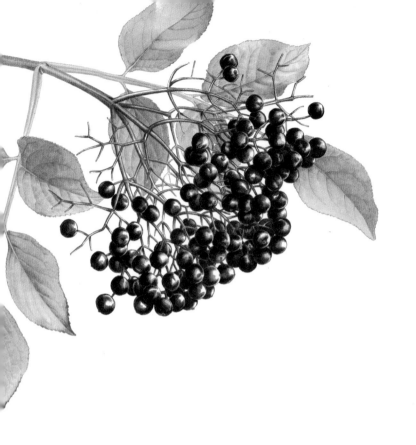

Colds & flu

*F*ALSTAFF:
What disease hast thou?

*B*ULLCALF:
A whoreson cold, sir, a cough, sir.

WILLIAM SHAKESPEARE,
King Henry IV, Part 2 (1597–98)

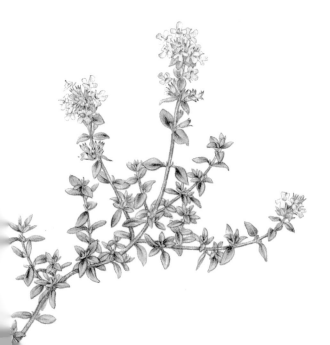

We all self-medicate when afflicted with colds and flu – if only a honey and lemon drink, or a menthol and eucalyptus lozenge. Honey will soothe a sore throat and is also expectorant, while strong-smelling compounds help to clear a blocked nose. We might buy over-the-counter remedies to reduce our temperature or relieve a headache, too. We might seek to strengthen our immune system, to avoid future illness. This is nothing new. Our ancestors disliked the misery of a cold just as much as we do, and used a variety of plants to relieve symptoms, hasten recovery and stave off further attacks. The Old English *Leechbook of Bald* gives many recipes to treat coughs, catarrh, *gesnote*, sore throats and even one for chapped lips.

❧ Boneset

Say 'boneset' to a British herbalist and they will immediately think of comfrey and its traditional importance in setting broken bones. Here we are talking about what American herbalists know as boneset: *Eupatorium perfoliatum*, a tall plant with pale, frothy flowerheads that commonly grows in damp places all over the eastern half of North America. Its other common names include 'thoroughwort' and 'ague-weed'. The Cherokee, Iroquois and others used an infusion of the aerial parts to treat colds and especially feverish flu, and it was quickly adopted by early settlers. Leaves and tops were gathered just as it came into flower, in late summer.

Although the Iroquois did make a poultice of it to treat fractures, boneset is said to have got its name because it was an effective treatment for a particularly nasty flu strain, which made you feel as though all your bones were breaking. Boneset was listed in the official US Pharmacopoeia, and was employed to good effect in several US flu epidemics in the nineteenth century. A hot infusion would promote therapeutic sweating, while drunk cold it was a tonic, stimulating the immune system. Though beware, as large doses have a laxative and emetic effect and could potentially be toxic, so please take medical advice to ensure you are taking an appropriate dose.

Eupatorium is a genus of plants named after Mithridates Eupator (120–63 BCE), a famous herbalist and King of Pontus (now in modern Turkey), who is supposed to have used a local species as an antidote to poison. Many Eupatorium species are native to the Americas, including Joe-pye weed or gravel root (Eupatorium – now Eutrochium – purpureum), with its vanilla-scented leaves. It is a diuretic and was prescribed to treat kidney stones and gravel. Our common European native Eupatorium cannabinum, the hemp agrimony (which is neither a hemp nor an agrimony), was historically given as a febrifuge (to drive away fever) but now, like many of its relatives, is grown mainly as an excellent nectar plant in wild gardens, attracting clouds of bees and butterflies.

✎ Echinacea

My neighbour, a hospital doctor, swears by echinacea when
she has a cold or flu. Starting the tablets at the first sign,
she says, relieves the symptoms and limits the duration
of the infection. Scientific studies support her assertion,
as does a mountain of anecdotal evidence. Various species
of echinacea are thought to be helpful for a variety of
conditions, especially for colds, flu and other infections
of the upper respiratory tract. The Cheyenne, for example,
chewed the root of Echinacea angustifolia to relieve a sore
throat, while the Choctaw did the same with Echinacea
purpurea for coughs. Echinacea angustifolia and Echinacea pallida
were both also used by Native Americans to cleanse and
heal wounds and burns, and to treat inflammations and
infections.

Echinaceas all originate in eastern and central North
America, but are now popular in gardens everywhere. They
are often included in 'prairie plantings', echoing their natural
habitat, and are excellent for attracting pollinating insects.
We know it as 'purple coneflower', from the cone-shaped
central boss of dark, spiky florets. Linnaeus gave the genus
its scientific name, from echinos, a Greek word for 'hedgehog'.
We most often grow varieties of Echinacea purpurea in our
gardens, for the striking summer flowers and handsome
winter seedheads. Its fresh roots were used medicinally in
the past, but most of the echinacea cold remedies sold today
are derived from its aerial parts.

In recent decades, echinacea has acquired a popular
reputation for enhancing the immune system. Research

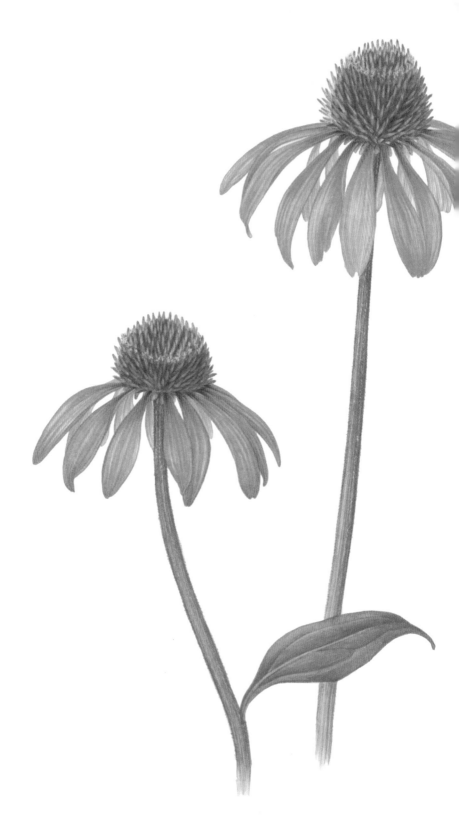

shows that it does in fact stimulate the production of white blood cells, which fight infection. It also contains a great deal of inulin, which is thought to encourage 'good bacteria' in the gut. However, taking echinacea long term is not recommended, and people with compromised immune systems should avoid it altogether. But I will quite happily reach for echinacea tablets whenever I notice that sore throat and stuffy nose.

∾ Thyme

Many of us grow thyme in our gardens for a constant supply of the fresh herb, and most of us have a tub of dried thyme in the store cupboard. There are many wild species of thyme and lots of garden varieties bred for their variegated leaves or slightly different aroma. All of them grow best in well-draining soil in a sunny position. Thyme is, as Theophrastus put it, 'patient of drought and, in general, needs moisture less [than other herbs]'. Some prostrate varieties will even thrive between paving stones, where they can be trodden on, releasing their characteristic fragrance. This aroma was supposed to impart courage and strength and, it is said, the Crusaders wore sprigs of it for that reason. Or perhaps they just wanted to smell better after months of travelling.

Theophrastus wrote that thyme was best propagated by division or cuttings, as the seed was invisible. Some even doubted that thyme seed existed at all, but Pliny

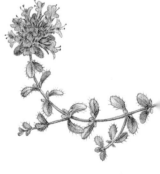

maintained that it must, so recommended planting the spent flowers. In fact, it has been estimated that there are 17,000 seeds to the ounce. Thyme grows wild in dry, rocky Mediterranean areas, attracting bees which make a delicious honey from its nectar. The most prized was Attic honey, made from thyme growing in the Hymettus mountains near Athens; so naturally, people did their best to transplant 'Attic thyme' to their own gardens. However, as Theophrastus noted, 'all the wild kinds [of herbs] are less juicy than the cultivated, and perhaps this is the very reason why most of them are more pungent and stronger'. Like many herbs, good thyme needs 'growing hard'.

Common thyme (Thymus vulgaris) originates in the western Mediterranean, but is now naturalised in Greece, too. It is the species most often grown in gardens and most often used in medicine or cooking, although other thymes are sometimes substituted. The commonest British native species, wild thyme (Thymus praecox subsp. Britannicus), also likes well-drained slopes. Poet John Clare, daydreaming about his beloved countryside, talked of 'where the wild thyme has cushioned mole-hills for a seat', and of course Titania's 'bank where the wild thyme blows' is familiar to us all. If you can't establish a thyme seat in your garden, you can easily grow thyme in pots. Although it flowers in summer, it is useful for cooking all year round, and for medicine particularly in the winter. Fortunately, thyme retains its fragrance very well when dried, so there is always the store-cupboard option, too.

On a home stay in the mountains of Armenia, we were given fresh thyme tea each evening after dinner. Our hostess told us it would help our digestion. *The Assyrian Herbal*, compiled from fragments of writings and tablets dating back to around 1000 BCE, records thyme being used to treat both breathing and digestive disorders, so the Armenian tradition has deep roots. The remains of a closely related species, *Thymbra spicata*, were found in Tutankhamun's tomb, possibly linked to the embalming process. Thymol, an essential oil found in thyme and some other plants, is a powerful antiseptic and disinfectant. The Sumerians used thyme as an antiseptic, and the ninth-century Iraqi physician al-Kindi treated bacterial infections with it. In France in 1868, two medical scientists advocated the use of thymol, instead of the more usual carbolic acid, as a disinfectant and for wound dressings. I should think it would at least have smelt better, though it is not recommended to apply undiluted thyme oil to the skin, or to take it internally at all. Thymol nowadays gives fragrance and flavour to many toothpastes, mouthwashes and gargles. Thyme is perfectly safe to eat in food, but medicinal doses should be avoided in pregnancy.

Since classical times, the main medicinal use of thyme has been in treating coughs and respiratory infections. Culpeper says: 'this herb is a notable strengthener of the lungs. It purges the body of phlegm, and is an excellent remedy for shortness of breath.' Modern research seems to bear this out. Several reputable, commercially available cough remedies contain thyme. When I have a cough, I supplement these remedies with cups of thyme tea sweetened with honey, as both are expectorant and taste good, too.

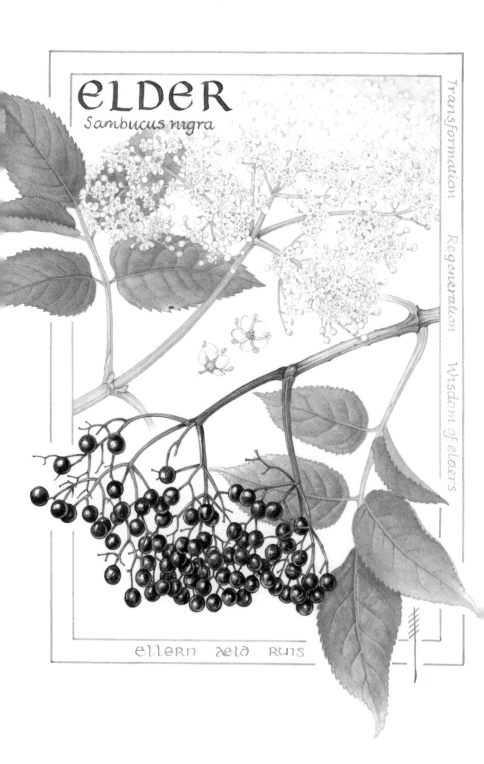

ELDER
Sambucus nigra

Transformation

Regeneration

Wisdom of elders

ellern aeld ruis

❧ Elder

It's so good in the middle of winter to think of high summer
hedgerows with elder bushes full of musky-smelling, creamy-
white blossoms, borne in flat-topped inflorescences like tea
plates. Like many families, we used to collect elderflowers
to make fritters, cordial and wine. My mother won prizes
for her delicate white elderflower wine, and for the red wine
she made from the berries that followed. I always pick and
freeze some flowers to add to gooseberry dishes, as they go
so well together. And elderflowers and berries both feature in
preparations to alleviate winter colds and flu.

Common elder (*Sambucus nigra*) is indeed very common
in hedgerows and on waste ground all over Europe, North
Africa and western Asia. There are related species in other
places: American elder (*Sambucus canadensis*) and blue elder
(*Sambucus cerulea*) were both used medicinally, though
American elder has poisonous roots. In Europe, elder
attracted a great deal of folklore, much of it contradictory.
It was favoured by witches; but growing by your door, would
protect the house from evil. It was said to be the tree from
which Judas hanged himself, though it hardly seems tall
enough or robust enough for that.

Folk medicine has always made use of elder, and it
features in all the old herbals, too. In 1644 an entire book
was published on its medical benefits and, twenty years later,
John Evelyn wrote that 'if the medicinal properties of the
leaves, bark, berries etc., were thoroughly known', everyone
could 'fetch a remedy from every hedge, either for sickness
or wound'.

Another country name for elder is 'boor-tree' meaning 'pipe tree'. Roman children are known to have hollowed out elder twigs to make flutes. In his 1870 diary, Francis Kilvert describes an elderly man temporarily curing his deafness by sticking an 'ellern twig' in his ear. Sticking anything in the ear is rather dangerous, but I wonder whether in fact the old man was using a hollow twig as a sort of ear-trumpet.

Common elder roots and bark were used in Hippocrates' time as powerful purgatives and emetics, thankfully abandoned now. Elder leaves, which Gerard called 'of a rank and stinking smell' were made into a good insecticidal spray for fruit trees, while sprigs of fresh leaves kept flies out of kitchens and dairies. Until the mid-twentieth century 'green elder ointment', made from the leaves simmered in lard, was a domestic remedy for bruises, wounds and piles. The parts most often used nowadays are the flowers and berries.

Elderflower water was listed in the official British Pharmacopoeia until at least the 1930s, mostly as a component in eye and skin preparations. It had a reputation for whitening and softening the skin. Several early Women's Institute books include recipes for face cream made with elderflowers simmered in lard or Vaseline. But elderflower is best known as a good, old-fashioned remedy for hay fever, sore throats, colds and catarrh. An infusion of the fresh or dried flowers will help especially with a feverish cold, as it promotes sweating.

By late summer, the flowers have developed into glossy black berries which are slightly toxic when raw – to humans, though not, apparently, to birds. Drying or cooking removes the toxicity, so, as long as the berries are handled with care,

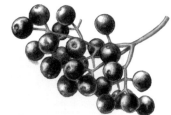

Elderberry rob

Wash the berries and strip them from the stems –
a fork is useful for this. Put them in a pan with
just enough water to cover. Bring to the boil, then
simmer gently for about half an hour, or until
they are soft.

Strain them to remove the bitter seeds.

Return the liquid to the pan and add 150g sugar
to every 250ml juice (about 5oz per ½ pint).
Heat and stir until the sugar dissolves.

Then boil briskly until it thickens to a syrupy
consistency – this can take just a few minutes, or
much longer, but take care it doesn't 'catch' or
burn.

When cooled, either pour into sterilised bottles and
seal the tops, or freeze in small containers or even
ice-cube trays.

Take a teaspoonful or two in a mug of hot water
last thing at night.

I also make a spicy version by adding a piece of
ginger, some cloves and a cinnamon stick along
with the sugar. Lovely drizzled over ice cream!

pies, jams and syrups should be perfectly safe. Elderberries had a reputation for helping with sciatica and rheumatic pain, and Mrs Grieve relates a story that supports this view: in 1899, an American sailor told a Prague physician that frequently getting drunk on port had cured his rheumatic pain. It turned out that he was drinking cheap port heavily adulterated with elderberry juice and that pure, genuine port had no effect. Experiments concluded that the most effective medicine consisted of 3 parts of elderberry juice to 1 part of port.

In the 1930s, my father's elderly maiden aunts, like generations before them, used to take hot elderberry wine at bedtime to treat colds and flu. Or they made a 'hot toddy' with elderberry 'rob' in a cup of hot water ('rob', first recorded in 1578, is an old word for a fruit syrup – see recipe on previous page). Blackberry or raspberry syrup can be made the same way, but elderberry is especially useful in winter. Recent research in Israel and Norway has shown that antioxidant elderberries contain a compound effective in preventing and treating several different strains of influenza.

Further reading

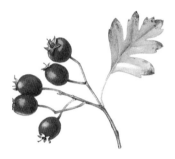

I f you have enjoyed what the ancient herbal writers had
to say, and would like to read more, here are a few ideas.
Many of the original texts are accessible in full online,
but more digestible editions of the foremost writers are
available in book form.

Pliny the Elder, *Natural History: A selection*, translated and
edited by John F. Healy, Penguin Classics. A great taste of Pliny's
huge range of interests in the natural world, these are highlights
from his monumental, 37-volume work *Natural History*.

John Gerard's masterly work *The Herbal, or General History of
Plants* has hardly ever been out of print since first published
in 1597. There are several modern editions, most of which
make selections from Thomas Johnson's 1636 edition of
Gerard. Many are illustrated with the original woodcuts, and
the plants are delightfully described in Gerard's scholarly but
engaging words.

Nicholas Culpeper's *Complete Herbal* is another perennial,
with many editions available. His encyclopaedic knowledge

is entertainingly written, and he is not afraid to voice his strong opinions, often very wittily.

There is such a bewildering variety of modern herbals for sale these days that it is hard to know which to choose. I would suggest checking that the author is an accredited herbalist, a member of a recognised professional organisation, and please remember that all remedies should be used with care.

Acknowledgements
& abbreviations

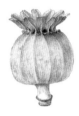

My thanks to all the friends who have helped, encouraged and supported me through the writing of this book, especially to Paul Harmes, FLS, for correcting my botanical blunders. Also to the wonderful team of kind and helpful editors at Yale University Press, London, for sparking the idea and steering me deftly through the publishing process. I am grateful to all the writers, herbalists, historians, storytellers, botanists, naturalists, countryfolk, cooks and others, whether contemporary or historical, from whom I have learned so much. Some of them are listed below.

QUOTED OR REFERRED TO FREQUENTLY THROUGH THE TEXT

Theophrastus, *Enquiry into Plants*, trans. Sir Arthur Hort (Loeb Classical Library 70), Harvard University Press, 1916

Pliny the Elder, *Natural History*, vols VI and VII, trans. W.H.S. Jones (Loeb Classical Library 392 and 393), Harvard University Press, 1951 and 1956

Leechbook of Bald, English, compiled in the tenth century, transcribed by C. Doyle, 2017

John Gerard, *The Herball, or General History of Plants*, London, 1597 edition

Nicholas Culpeper, *The English Physician*, London, 1652 edition

Maud Grieve, *A Modern Herbal*, Jonathan Cape, 1931

Sarah E. Edwards, Ines da Costa Rocha, Elizabeth M. Williamson and Michael Heinrich, *Phytopharmacy: An Evidence-based Guide to Herbal Medicinal Products*, Wiley Blackwell, 2015

INTRODUCTION

Laurie Lee, *Cider with Rosie*, Hogarth Press, 1959

Anthony Huxley, *Green Inheritance*, Gaia Books, 1984

FOODS AS MEDICINE

Figs – reference from L.P. Maenu'u, *An Indicative List of Solomon Islands Medicinal Plants*, unpublished, 1979 (courtesy of Dr M. Clark)

SPRING

Celandine – Richard Mabey, *Flora Britannica*, Chatto & Windus, 1996

Coltsfoot – Sir John Clerk, from his unpublished Diary, 'Clerk of Penicuik Papers', Scottish Records Office GD 18/2412, quoted in Gabrielle Hatfield, *Memory, Wisdom and Healing*, The History Press, 1999

Docks – Channel Island proverb quoted in Gabrielle Hatfield, *Memory, Wisdom and Healing*, The History Press, 1999

EARLY SUMMER

Balm – Dioscorides, *De Materia Medica*, trans. Tess Anne Osbaldeston, Ibidis, 2000
Poppies – An extract from 'Big Poppy', from Ted Hughes, *Collected Poems*, Faber & Faber Ltd, 2005, p. 724, reproduced by permission of the publisher and Farrar, Straus & Giroux, LLC, all rights reserved

HIGH SUMMER

Manuscript of Benediktbeuern, in Helen Waddell (trans.), *Mediaeval Latin Lyrics*, Penguin, 1929
Lavender – from an old family recipe book, c.1790, quoted in a Devon Women's Institute cookery book (no date)

AUTUMN

Blackberries (dewberries) – T. Woollgar, *Flora Lewensis*, unpublished manuscript (1790–1809), Brighton and Hove City Libraries
Fennel – Hildegard von Bingen, *Physica*, trans. Priscilla Throop, Healing Arts Press, 1998

WINTER

Ginger – Dioscorides, *De Materia Medica*, trans. Tess Anne Osbaldeston, Ibidis, 2000

Marigold – Sir John Clerk, from his unpublished Diary, 'Clerk of Penicuik Papers', Scottish Records Office GD 18/2412, quoted in Gabrielle Hatfield, *Memory, Wisdom and Healing*, The History Press, 1999

Sloes – rhyme quoted in H.E. Corke and G.C. Nuttall, *Wild Flowers as They Grow*, Cassell & Co., 1912

ABBREVIATIONS

cv	cultivar
sp	species (singular)
spp	species (plural)
var	variety

Index

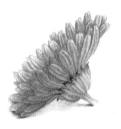

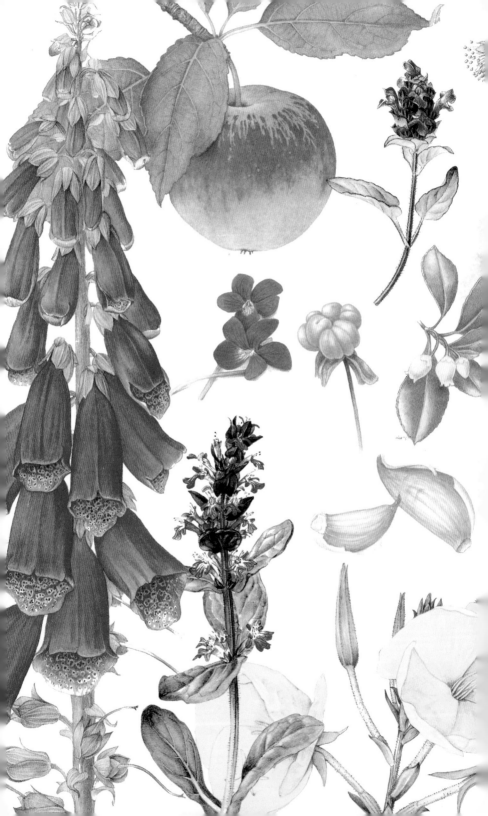